Advance Reader Praise for *The Religion of Thinness*

"Michelle Lelwica has written a truly transformative book. It represents a call for women to band together to help them finally break free from the cult-like Religion of Thinness and take back their lives."
— **Marion A. Bilich, PhD**, coauthor of *Shared Grace: Therapists and Clergy Working Together*

"This is an accessible and important book that offers both theory and practice for women who want to free themselves from the pervasive obsession with body projects. The author's voice is mature and acutely critical of the ways in which American culture embraces thinness and its pursuit as a form of religion."
— **Joan Jacobs Brumberg, PhD**, author of *Fasting Girls* and *The Body Project*

"We have known, on some level, that a 'Religion of Thinness' is lurking in our lives but in her book, Lelwica brilliantly points out its dogma, churches, evangelists, bibles, and hymns. Furthermore, readers are offered 'a way out' of the usual indoctrination with suggestions for antidotes, support, and deprogramming. *The Religion of Thinness* will be an addition to my 'must read' list for colleagues and clients."
— **Carolyn Costin, MFT**, Clinical Director, Monte Nido, Malibu, CA, and author of *The Eating Disorder Sourcebook* and *100 Questions and Answers about Eating Disorders*

"This book should be required reading. We have believed for so long that there is only one kind of beauty, only one 'perfect' body, and have similarly come to believe that our disordered attitudes toward food are actually normal. They are not. Lelwica overturns these assumptions, asking us to examine our long-held faith in the tragic Religion of Thinness, and opens the door to a new way of being in our bodies and in the world."
— **Marya Hornbacher**, author of *Wasted* and *Madness*

"This is a profoundly meaningful, elegantly-written book designed to cultivate a certain cultural and media literacy that can enhance spiritual growth and awaken us to our true hungers. I highly recommend it to women seeking freedom from food issues and dieting—and to all who desire a life that is spiritually rich and fulfilling."

   – **Anita Johnston, PhD**, author of *Eating in the Light of the Moon*

"An important and original contribution to the field. Lelwica expertly shows how our worship of thinness masks a much deeper spiritual need and leaves us starving for meaning and purpose in our lives. By providing a wide variety of practical ways to nourish our bodies and spirits, she offers real hope and inspiration."

   – **Jean Kilbourne, EdD**, creator of the film series "Killing Us Softly," author of *Can't Buy My Love*, and Senior Scholar, Wellesley Centers for Women

"Through a thoughtful, comprehensive critique of the religious, gender-based, and cultural factors that brainwash women to be pro-thin and anti-fat, Lelwica gently guides the reader to question body hatred and the quest for body perfection. Moreover, she provides a way out of women's obsession with thinness—through body and emotional mindfulness and critical assessment of cultural messages—that will bring them true inner peace and happiness."

   – **Karen R. Koenig, LCSW, MEd**, author of *The Rules of "Normal" Eating* and *The Food and Feelings Workbook*

"An inspiring and timely work, *The Religion of Thinness* illustrates how contemporary women have come to mistake the community of dieting, weight loss, and disordered eating with true, soul-satisfying connections and spiritual salvation. This well-written, thought-provoking book offers a spiritual paradigm that might really save our souls—and our bodies!"

   – **Margo Maine, PhD, FAED**, author of *Father Hunger* and *Body Wars*

"Lelwica describes how the culture of 'more' can be replaced by a culture of gratitude and care for one's body. The book examines and criticizes media messages, but it also provides exercises that can re-orient mind and body from self-disparaging and destructive attitudes to healthful and life giving ideas and practices. This is a wonderful book, well researched and accessible. *The Religion of Thinness* will be a godsend to anyone who wants to exchange a 'religion' constructed by American media for more life-enhancing values."

— **Margaret R. Miles, PhD**, author and former Bussey Professor of Theology at the Harvard University Divinity School

"Michelle Lelwica's reflections are revelatory and her call to mind-fulness is inviting and creative. Not only does she reveal why so many thousands of women have abdicated their power to the Religion of Thinness, she lays out a plan for returning to one's authentic spiritual center. This book is truly food for the soul!"

— **Jan Phillips**, author of *The Art of Original Thinking* and *Divining the Body*

"Stop battling your body, and fill your life with connection, balance, and joy. With a focus on mindfulness and cultural criticism, including real advertisements to analyze the media's true message, Lelwica teaches the reader to question society's superficial ideals. Her concept of form-ing communities to discuss these topics is brilliant! It is a must-read for men and women of all ages!"

— **Jenni Schaefer**, author of *Life Without Ed* and *Goodbye Ed, Hello Me*

"By using the premise that the pursuit of the 'perfect' body has be-come a religion in today's society, Lelwica is able to delve deeply into the connection between body, health, and spirituality, while also offer-ing ways to combat the superficiality of focusing solely on one's outer appearance. This thoughtful, well-researched book is a great addition to the literature on eating disorders and related issues."

— **Jess Weiner**, Self-esteem expert and author of *A Very Hungry Girl* and *Life Doesn't Begin 5 Pounds from Now*

"With the publication of this outstanding new book, Dr. Michelle Lelwica has created a wise, practical, and dynamic resource for all individuals on their journey to recovery from eating and body image problems. Lelwica's grasp of the spiritual issues that perplex human beings in the 21st Century is matched only by her ability to communicate her depth of understanding in a stimulating, clear, and effective manner. I will recommend this remarkable book to patients and family members whose lives have been impacted by an eating disorder and urge other clinicians to do the same."

– **Kathryn Zerbe, MD**, author of *The Body Betrayed* and *Integrated Treatment of Eating Disorders*

"Lelwica doesn't want readers to merely observe the parallels between worshipping a deity and worshipping thinness, she wants readers to find personal satisfaction through other means. The myths, rituals, images, and moral codes of the Religion of Thinness are explored, and readers are encouraged to think critically about these elements and practice more mindful behaviors. Clearly, Lelwica hopes to turn around the statistics with which she begins the book; *The Religion of Thinness* helps to wake readers to thinness' false promises, and it pushes them to seek a salvation built on more solid ground."

– **Jessica Higgins**, *ForeWord Magazine*

"In this thought-provoking narrative, Lelwica considers the obsession with thinness in the context of the broader cultural, religious, and historical influences on women's attitudes toward weight and food. She then offers components of healing that can lead to a fuller, more satisfying life."

– *Library Journal*

THE RELIGION OF THINNESS

The

RELIGION *of* THINNESS

Satisfying the Spiritual Hungers behind Women's Obsession with Food and Weight

MICHELLE M. LELWICA, THD

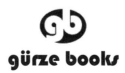

gürze books

The Religion of Thinness
Satisfying the Spiritual Hungers behind Women's Obsession with Food and Weight

© 2010 by Michelle M. Lelwica, ThD

Gürze Books, LLC
P.O. Box 2238
Carlsbad, CA 92018
(800) 756-7533
www.gurze.com

Cover design by Rob Johnson, Toprotype, Mt. Pleasant, SC
Author photo: Lisa Gingerich

Library of Congress Cataloging-in-Publication Data

Lelwica, Michelle Mary.
The religion of thinness : satisfying the spiritual hungers behind women's obsession with food and weight / Michelle M. Lelwica.
p. cm.
Includes bibliographical references and index.
ISBN 978-0-936077-55-0
1. Eating disorders--Patients--Religious life. 2. Women--Health and hygiene--Religious aspects. I. Title.
RC552.E18L437 2010
362.196'8526--dc22
2009035748

Disclaimers:

The authors and publishers of this book intend for this publication to complement, not substitute for, any professional medical and/or psychological services.

When quotes reflect the statements of actual persons, they are always referenced. However, anonymous quotations are from composite characters based on the author's experiences with real women.

First Edition

1 3 5 7 9 0 8 6 4 2

FOR ROBERT, ANTHONY, AND GIULIO

Table of Contents

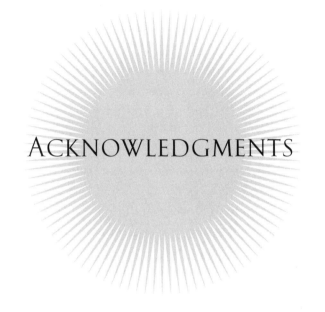

ACKNOWLEDGMENTS

My desire for women of every size, shape, color, and culture to feel at home in their bodies is a great source of meaning in my life, one that grows out of my journey of learning to respect, nurture, appreciate, and enjoy my own body. Many people have supported me along the way, particularly in the process of writing this book. It gives me great pleasure to thank some of them here.

Cissy Brady-Rogers is the one who urged me to write a book about religion, spirituality, and eating disorders for a popular audience. For several years, we worked on earlier drafts of *The Religion of Thinness* together. Cissy not only helped with editing, but also contributed substantive insights. As a therapist who incorporates a spiritual perspective into her work with women with eating problems, she generously offered invaluable practical ideas, including the concept of "practicing peace with your body," which she coined. Through her workshops, writings, and clinical work, she has enriched the lives of so many women. I am deeply grateful to her for extending the wisdom of her experience and expertise to readers of this book.

My publishers at Gürze Books, Lindsey and Leigh Cohn, believed in the project throughout its long gestation period. It would be hard to overstate how much heart, sweat, and intelligence they put into its development. Both of them read and edited the manuscript countless times. When the writing process seemed never-ending, Lindsey's undying enthusiasm lifted my spirits. Over the years, she shared with me her knowledge about eating disorders, her skills as an author, and her keen and compassionate understanding of the human spirit. As the chapters got closer to being finished, Leigh volunteered endless hours to comb through them (again), working on weekends and late in the evening to improve the writing and enhance the content. Without his heroic help and endurance, *The Religion of Thinness* would have never been born. I am forever grateful to both Lindsey and Leigh not only for their essential contributions to this book, but also for the friendship we formed in the process of working together.

The other person whose assistance was pivotal to the book's completion is Spencer Smith, a professional writer and also a good friend. Spencer's job was to help me translate my ideas for readers outside the academy. In this process, he shared his talent for accessible writing as well as his intuitive understanding of this book's message. He grasped immediately both the importance of challenging our culture's obsession with thinness and the need for women to find more healthy ways to nourish their bodies and spirits. To that end, he helped develop the book's practical exercises to complement its more theoretical ideas. Ultimately, both the passion and the know-how Spencer brought to this book helped convince me of its importance and inspired me to stick with it.

Within academia, I would like to thank my friends and colleagues at Concordia College, whose sharp intellects and immense hearts gave me the assurances I needed to write outside of my academic comfort zone. In particular, I am grateful to Dr. Roy Hammerling (my Department Chair) and Dr. James Aageson (my Dean) for their humble style of leadership. Others in the Religion Department—especially Professor Hilda Koster, Dr. Jan Pranger, and Dr. Shawn Carruth—were a constant source of sanity and strength as I sought to juggle my academic and family responsibilities with my desire to finish this book. Dr. Ahmed Afzaal helped with several of the book's examples from Islam; Ms. Mary Thornton assisted by printing, copying, and mailing drafts at various stages; and Ms. Emma Hoglund helped with some of the research for Chapters 6 and 7. To these and other Concordia friends and colleagues too numerous to mention, I am profoundly indebted. I also want to thank the hundreds of students I have had the privilege to teach both at Concordia College in Moorhead and at Saint Mary's College of California. Many of them have told me about their struggles with food and body image, and in doing so they have reminded me of the importance of the issues addressed in this book.

Through the years, a few close friends outside the academy—especially Theresa Traynor, Anne McGeary Snowdon, and Julia Freedgood—have supported my quest for personal and social transformation. Each in her own way has helped me remember what really matters in life, and that healing is a process. Their non-judgmental character and bottomless love have nurtured me over time and despite distance.

Finally, I would like to thank my family for all they have done, directly and indirectly, to help me stay grounded. My brothers and sister—Mark, Jim, John, and Sue Lelwica—along with their spouses and children, have always shown me the kind of unconditional acceptance that a human being needs to flourish. My parents in particular have had unshakable confidence in me and in my ability to write this book. They have spent weeks taking care of my children to give me time to work on it. I could not imagine navigating the vicissitudes of the writing process—much less my life—without their steady stream of support. And it is really them I have to thank for teaching me the importance of spiritual growth. Their own deep and dynamic faith has given me an example for a lifetime.

And to my husband, Robert Angotti, and our two beautiful sons, Giulio and Anthony, I have nothing but love and gratitude for all you have sacrificed to make this book possible. Thank you, Bobby, for enduring my moodiness at times when I wondered whether it would ever be done; and for the conversations we had related to different chapters, which always challenged me to think more carefully and clearly; and for the ways you encouraged me to take a break from my head and enjoy my life. Anthony and Giulio, you have been my greatest teachers when it comes to the art of living in the present. I'm forever thankful for the times you've urged me to turn off the computer and read you a story or head to the playground. You have given me more joy than you'll ever know.

INTRODUCTION

We live in a culture that worships thinness.

Americans spend over $60 billion per year trying to shed their "excess" flesh. Sales for weight loss products—from appetite suppressants to home delivered diet foods—are steadily on the rise. We are constantly bombarded with TV commercials and infomercials, Internet spam and banners, radio and print media advertisements—all peddling ways to help us tighten and trim. Marketing gurus in the book-publishing industry refer to January as "New Year New You"—walk into any bookstore franchise during this critical sales season and you'll find it stacked with titles designed to help you lose weight, look "great," and live "right." Perhaps not surprisingly, diet books outsell any other books on the market—except the Bible.[1]

The weight-loss industry is, however, only part of the picture.

Need to buy groceries? You can't miss the "women's magazines" at the checkout counter. The cover of almost every one depicts a celebrity or model that both defines and is defined by a very narrow and relatively precise paradigm of female beauty. She is tall (maybe 5'10"), slender (about 110 pounds), and her body is meticulously toned. She is often a Barbie-type: white, blue-eyed, and blond-haired, although this long-standing tradition is shifting to include more women of color. Alongside these "beautiful" (skinny) women are the familiar headlines: "Lose 10 Pounds in 10 Days," "Fight Flab! Look Fab!"—or some variation on this monotonous theme. And, if you get bored staring at the collage of fat-free beauties while you're waiting to pay for your groceries, you can always look at the *un*flattering pictures of these same women in tabloids with accusatory headlines about any extreme weight gain or loss.

Media images establish what it means to be a beautiful woman in our society. It doesn't matter that the vast majority of us don't look like the women we are taught to adore. In fact, that's part of the ploy: the relative rarity of the "ideal" creates tremendous pressure for ordinary women to "improve" their appearance. Weight-loss is essential to this transformation, or so we are told with both words and pictures. And the more we come to believe this truth, the more we absorb other messages as well—ones that are less obvious (and perhaps more insidious for being so), but no less powerful. These messages teach us that our souls will only feel as good as our bodies look; that we can never be happy unless we strive for physical perfection; and that to be successful, loved, and satisfied, we must try to emulate the images we have come to idolize.

Little wonder that in this cultural milieu, the numbers of undergraduate women with eating and body image problems are skyrocketing. Some studies have shown that up to 20 percent of college women suffer from an eating disorder.[2] Another found that 40 percent of college women showed "anorexic-like" behavior—nearly half of them engaged in bingeing and purging—and all of them knew someone else with similarly-disordered behaviors.[3] Another study discovered that a third of college women surveyed reported using "diet aids" in the past 12 months, including diet pills, fat blockers, diuretics, and laxatives.[4] There have even been reports of plumbing problems in dormitories due to widespread vomiting.[5] Binge eating without purging is more common than anorexia and bulimia combined.[6] One survey found that 67 percent of college women binge-eat.[7]

These behaviors are extremely debilitating—if not deadly. Anorexia nervosa has the highest mortality rate of any psychiatric illness,[8] and survivors often spend months in the hospital and years in treatment.

However, anorexia, bulimia, and binge eating are only one part of a broad continuum of difficulties women have with food, weight, and body image.

How many times have you tried to lose weight? How many hours have you spent preoccupied with the size of your waist, hips, or thighs?

If your answer is "too many," you are hardly alone. More than three-quarters of healthy-weight adult women in the U.S. believe they are "too fat," and nearly two-thirds of high school girls are on diets.[9] Attempts to lose weight start very young: 80 percent of 4th grade girls surveyed said they had already been on diets. The same percentage of women in their mid-50s express a desire to be thinner.[10] Meanwhile, growing numbers of women of color are joining the ranks of those who chronically hate their bodies, and more and more men are worrying about the "spare tire" around their midriffs or the layer of flesh that sags from their chins.[11]

Many people spend a lifetime struggling with their weight. Why? Is it really to fend off the health-related dangers we hear so much about and have come to fear? To be sure, the physical ailments that some studies link to excess weight—heart disease, diabetes, and certain types of cancer—are well known and cause for alarm. Indeed, many of us are more prone to eat too much and exercise too little than to over-abstain or exercise excessively. But, weight-loss is a precarious strategy for "getting fit," especially in light of the growing evidence suggesting that thinner is not *necessarily* healthier. Some studies raise questions about whether being moderately overweight is automatically unhealthy and whether it should be treated at all.[12] In fact, research verifies that, like happiness and beauty, health is possible in a wide variety of shapes and sizes.[13] In the end, health risks may have less to do with our drive for thinness than other, less tangible factors.

* * *

I propose that our obsessions with eating and weight mask the deeper needs of our spirits. We are looking for a way to maintain peace, order, and security in a world that seems out of control. We want to be happy and healthy, to feel accepted and connected within a larger community. We need to sense that our lives are meaningful—that we have a greater purpose.

The traditional way to manage these kinds of spiritual yearnings has been through religion. In the west, Christianity has been the predominant faith since the 4th century. However, in today's world, the authority of Christianity, as well as other organized religions, is contested and in some ways declining.[14] This has made it possible for women in our culture to break out of the constraining roles they had been kept in for so long, but it has also created a vacuum, a feeling that something is missing. The need for meaningful symbols, beliefs, stories, and rituals by which to organize our lives and understand our purpose has not disappeared. In fact, we are starving for them.

In an attempt to fill this void, many women have adopted what I call "The Religion of Thinness." This "religion" teaches us that controlling our weight will give us a feeling of control over our lives. It offers us the hope of health and happiness through the idea of the "perfect" body, which we believe is attainable through diet and exercise. It teaches us to feel morally superior if we "eat right" (meaning fewer fat grams or calories), and connects us to a larger community of women who are trying to lose weight. It gives us rituals—like counting and burning calories—that create a sense of order. And it includes a plethora of icons and symbols in the form of models and actresses in whose image we are encouraged to recreate ourselves. Perhaps most importantly of all, it gives us an ultimate purpose—the "salvation" that comes from being thin.

But in the end its promises are hollow. The Religion of Thinness cannot fill the emptiness we feel inside ourselves. It cannot satisfy our deepest hungers. The hope it offers is an illusion, one that we have been fed by the media and other sources, and one that many of us have consumed with a religious-like fervor in our quest for meaning and purpose.

I know, because I too was once a disciple.

* * *

When I was starving and bingeing and purging some 30 years ago, I didn't have a name for what I was doing. I knew that more than anything else I wanted to be thin, but I had no idea where this desire came from, much less the extent to which others shared my passion. It wasn't until I learned of the death of Karen Carpenter, the 32-year-old pop singer who died of heart failure in 1983 as a result of anorexia nervosa, that I started to worry about my weight-loss tactics. By then, I was no longer spending entire days looking for opportunities to gorge and vomit, but I was still preoccupied with food and just as hell-bent on getting skinny.

Much has changed since those days. When it comes to eating problems, anorexia and bulimia have become household words. Children and grandparents alike understand their meanings. And, during the past few decades, the desire to be thinner has increased dramatically and become more stubbornly entrenched in the hearts and minds of an even wider variety of people. These days I would be diagnosed with an eating disorder. When I was growing up I called it "dieting."

Like so many girls and women today, the prospect of thinness consumed me for much of my adolescence. Never mind that I was born with the short, round, and relatively soft body of my Polish and Swiss-German ancestors. Even though I was at a healthy weight according to the doctor's charts, I wanted to be thinner, more angular. I wanted my bones to protrude so that people would wonder how I could possibly have so much self-control and whether it hurt to be so hungry. I wanted people to notice me, to stare at me in amazement. I wanted them to see in my thin body an expression of my inner goodness.

Although I did not think of my dieting strategies in traditional religious terms, I was certain that God "Himself" was pleased whenever I denied my seemingly-constant urge to eat. Sometimes I would sit in church, praying for the strength to eat only the calories I had allotted myself that day. I would study other girls as they walked up the aisle to receive communion to determine whether I was fatter or thinner than they, and by implication whether I was inferior or superior in the eyes of God and others.

To further inspire my quest for the holiness of thinness, I read *Seventeen* magazine like a Bible, trying many of the slimming tips it offered—some of them to the extreme. I drank enormous quantities of water before meals to make myself too full to eat. I stayed up late at night doing hundreds of leg-lifts. I studied the caloric content of every food imaginable and measured the "success" of my days by how many or how few calories I ended up ingesting. I drank cups of vinegar because I thought the burn it caused in my chest and stomach meant that it was literally burning calories (it wasn't). All the while, I understood the physical discomfort of these bizarre rituals as proof that I was on the right track. Somehow the pain confirmed I was good.

I no longer have an eating disorder and I no longer believe that my happiness and worth depend on being skinny. Thoughts of my own body have shifted from loathing to gratitude and enjoyment. I now feel the life energy within my body and try to cultivate awareness of and appreciation for that vitality by caring for it lovingly. These days, I derive a sense of purpose not from trying to make my body thinner, but from being a mother, a wife, a daughter, and a global citizen, and from the work I do as college professor and scholar of religion. Even more fundamentally, I find meaning in my effort to use the various experiences I have in life—whether good or bad, stressful or soothing, predictable or surprising, or something in between—as opportunities to wake up, to open and expand my heart, and to be present to my life and the lives of others in ways that bring peace and healing.

When I tell people that I am a scholar in the field of religion and then mention my interest in eating disorders, many are initially confused. *How does religion relate to eating disorders?*

* * *

I explore this question throughout this book, along with some of the reasons we are experiencing a spiritual vacuum in our culture, and why so many women are devoting themselves to thinness to fill the void it has created. I will explain what The Religion of Thinness is, how its symbols, beliefs, rituals, and rules function, why it has gained so much traction in our culture, and how it has come to attract so many devotees. I will also explore how the mass media has helped establish this "religion" through its iconography of model women and by promoting negative and confusing images about food, weight, and appearance.

While a few books offer spiritual perspectives on women's preoccupation with eating and thinness, *The Religion of Thinness* considers this obsession in light of the broader cultural, religious, and historical influences on women's attitudes towards weight and food. Understanding these wider influences is crucial, because otherwise, eating problems are primarily seen as personal issues—an individual woman's failure to achieve the goals set forth by society. When the shame that many of us feel about our bodies is viewed in isolation, it obscures the cultural influences on our struggles with weight and eating. Whether they come in the form of compulsive eating, anorexia nervosa, bulimia, or simply a preoccupation with the scale, eating disorders are *social* problems, not personal failures. Indeed, they are rational responses to a culture that demands we be thin, not pathological responses to personal insults and injuries. They hook us by providing temporary relief from the suffering and insecurity that are part of the human condition.

Because of our culture's glorification of thinness, many of us spend incalculable energy wishing we were leaner, restricting our eating, and loathing ourselves when we don't succeed. For some, it's impossible to imagine what life would be like if we never had to worry about calories or give another thought to the size of our thighs. Many of us police our bodies with the kind of rigor only the most dangerous criminals require. Whether or not we realize it, our everyday feelings of dissatisfaction take a tremendous toll on us. Some of us obsess so much that there is little energy left for the creative work of our lives. Before we know it, our desire to minimize our bodies has inadvertently diminished our spirits.

The unfortunate truth is that by placing our hopes on the size of our bodies, we bury the deeper yearnings that are disguised by our anxieties about weight and eating, including a sense of purpose, inspiration, transformation, responsibility, unconditional love, and peace. The real problem is not our soft bellies or well-rounded buttocks. We crave much more than food, which is why some of us feel we can never get enough.

As long as we believe that the trouble resides in the amount of our flesh and act as though eating or starving is the answer to our insatiable hunger, we will miss the opportunity for inner work and personal growth that our eating problems present.

Recognizing our unmet spiritual needs is a crucial step toward freedom from perpetual angst about our bodies. This process requires us to be honest with ourselves and to muster the courage to face our problems squarely. Dwelling in the false hope that being skinny will make us happier, prettier, more successful, and free is like living in a dream. The freedom we long for demands that we see through these empty promises, while exploring the spiritual needs that led us to buy into such illusions in the first place.

The Religion of Thinness is designed to wake us up—not only to our spiritual longings but also to the ways we have been brainwashed into believing that our bodies are flawed and our appetites sinful. It examines the widespread cultural messages that contribute to the alienation so many women feel towards their bodies, and it urges readers to become critical of these messages. It also encourages us to identify the spiritual needs that are hidden within our desire to be thinner and to find more nourishing ways to address these needs.

* * *

This is a self-help book designed to foster readers' cultural critique and spiritual growth. It does this by offering two primary tools for awakening from the toxic cultural messages around us and becoming more deeply aware of the experience of our bodies and minds right *now*.

The first of these tools is the practice of *mindfulness*. To be mindful is to be fully aware of what is happening in your thoughts, feelings, body, and in the world around you in the present moment. It is a method of nonjudgmentally observing these things instead of identifying yourself with them. By increasing your awareness of what you are experiencing at any given moment, mindfulness enables you to be honest about what is really going on. Despite its Buddhist origins, mindfulness is essentially a practical skill that can be developed by persons of any spiritual background (including agnostics and atheists).

Learning to watch (rather than identify with) your inner experience helps you realize that you are not defined by your ideas. This means that you are not defined by all of the thoughts and feelings you have adopted regarding food, weight loss, and how you're "supposed" to look. Your life is rooted in something larger than that. Mindfulness practice has the power to put you in touch with this "something larger," reconnect you to your deepest values, and enable you to heal from the suffering your eating problems have created. Learning to be mindful can help you identify and address some of the spiritual needs that The Religion of Thinness obscures.

The second tool for recovery is *cultural criticism,* a technique that involves carefully examining the messages you receive from our culture about food and body image. I demonstrate this practice throughout the book by deconstructing and analyzing specific examples from contemporary media and by teaching you a set of skills that will empower you to do the same. I want you to recognize the *real* messages they are sending us, not the messages their corporate sponsors would have us blindly believe.

In a society that encourages us to "save" ourselves by shrinking our bodies, both cultural criticism and spiritual growth are integral aspects of our overall health and well-being. My hope is that the practices of mindfulness and cultural criticism I offer in this book will help you to challenge the authority of The Religion of Thinness and find new ways to satisfy the spiritual hungers beneath your obsession with food and weight loss.

* * *

The goal of this book is not to offer a "cure" or a "how to" method for recovering from eating problems. Rather, it is to change our mindset by presenting a different way of thinking about weight and eating. In this regard, I offer suggestions for *practicing peace with your body.* This is a phrase that therapist Cissy Brady-Rogers—who helped with the writing of this book—uses in her work with women who suffer from eating problems. It means learning how to accept your body just as it is and treat it with loving kindness, instead of trying to control, punish, or diminish it through endless dieting. This process is integral to healing the body hatred that so many of us have endured for so long.

The Religion of Thinness is for *anyone* who has struggled with body image and unwanted eating patterns—from people who are plagued by those "extra" 10 pounds, to those who starve, binge, and purge. Although I recognize that men increasingly find themselves facing similar challenges, as do people from cultures around the globe, it focuses primarily on the struggles of contemporary American girls and women.

I wrote this book because I know that challenging our culture's devotion to slenderness and addressing the spiritual needs that draw us to it are essential components of healing—healing that can lead to a life full of peace, love, compassion, courage, responsibility, and meaning. For when our spiritual hungers are well-fed, our bodies can become a source of joy rather than danger. When we find healthy outlets for our passions, eating and starving are no longer the center of our existence. When we find creative ways to attend to our desires, dilemmas, and disappointments, food and body are no longer the main source of our life's purpose. Instead, they become enjoyable parts of a truly meaningful life.

1

CHANGING THE PARADIGM

From "The Religion of Thinness" to Practicing Peace with Our Bodies

There is a more ominous hunger, and I was and am not alone in sensing it. It squirms under the sternum, clawing at the throat. At school we were hungry and lost and scared and young and we needed religion, salvation—something to fill the anxious hollow in our chests. Many of us sought it in food and thinness.

– Marya Hornbacher[1]

Our obsession with the "ideal" female body has grown to proportions that have never before been seen in the history of Western culture. Perhaps there is no better example of the extremes to which some women will go to achieve the "perfect body" and the underlying needs revealed by this obsession than in the relatively new and growing cyberspace subculture known as "Pro-Ana."

At the center of this Internet-driven underworld is the goddess "Ana" (short for *anorexia*) who is depicted as a fairy-like young woman with silken blond curls, glimmering white skin, and an ethereal, skeletal body. Among her devotees, Ana represents the epitome of feminine perfection, combining self-sacrifice and control with submission and self-loathing, all packaged in a frame that is quintessentially thin. On any given day, untold numbers of young women log on to Ana websites in search of *thinspiration*. The worldview of this new movement is encapsulated in the "Ana Creed":

> *I believe in Control, the only force mighty enough to bring order to the chaos that is my world.*

> *I believe that I am the most vile, worthless and useless person ever to have existed on the planet, and that I am totally unworthy of anyone's time and attention.*

> *I believe that other people who tell me differently are idiots. If they could see how I really am, then they would hate me almost as much as I do.*

> *I believe in perfection and strive to attain it.*

> *I believe in salvation through trying just a bit harder than I did yesterday.*

> *I believe in bathroom scales as an indicator of my daily successes and failures.*

> *I believe in hell, because I sometimes think that I am living in it.*

> *I believe in a wholly black and white world, the losing of weight, recrimination for sins, abnegation of the body and a life ever fasting.*[2]

In addition to the Ana Creed, the Ana subculture includes Ana prayers, an Ana Psalm, thinspirational images (e.g., photos of extremely thin models, celebrities, and actresses), Ana bracelets, The Thin Commandments, and moonlight rituals. Followers of Ana believe that anorexia and bulimia are lifestyle choices, rather than illnesses, and that people who go to extremes for the sake of thinness need not be bothered by the mediocre standards of ordinary people who simply cannot understand.[3] The members of this group celebrate their weight-loss achievements and support each other in their tireless efforts to bring order out of chaos by making their bodies disappear.

However troubling the Pro-Ana phenomenon may be, it's not altogether surprising. In many ways, its philosophy and practices are nothing but an extreme version of behaviors and beliefs that have become deeply woven into the fabric of mainstream American culture. Many people who don't have eating disorders identify with the attitudes and actions of those who do. You need not suffer from full-blown bulimia to measure your success by how much you weigh. You need not be all-out anorexic to use dieting as a means for gaining control. You need not be identified as obese to feel ashamed of your size or shape.

The perspectives and practices of Ana's disciples differ in *degree*, not in *kind*, from the thinking and habits of many "average" girls and women. In fact today, women, and increasing numbers of men, are encouraged as never before to equate their personal achievements, happiness, and sense of peace and security with the size of their bodies. Maybe you don't believe in the "recrimination of sins, the abnegation of the body, and life ever fasting" as the Pro-Anas do, but how much of your life have you spent judging your success or failure by the numbers you see on the bathroom scale? And how often have you viewed yourself as worthless or unlovable when your body showed signs of "imperfection"?

Perhaps you are one of an estimated 10 million women or 1 million men in the U.S. who suffer from an eating disorder.[4] Or maybe you are one of the many millions more who struggle with food, eating, dieting, body image, and weight concerns. If you are female, chances are you fall somewhere on a *continuum* of eating and body image problems, which range from the obviously disturbed behaviors such as starving, bingeing, and purging, to the less blatant but still crippling preoccupation with counting calories and eating-for-thinness, to the virtually omnipresent and seemingly normal desire to lose a few pounds.

Recognizing a continuum of conflicts related to weight and eating is important for several reasons. The vast number of women who find themselves somewhere on this continuum reveals the extent to which we live in a culture of disordered eating. By locating the root of the insanity in cultural norms and institutions (rather than individuals), a continuum model lessens the stigma attached to anorexia, bulimia, and related problems. At the same time, it empowers us to challenge a society that praises women for monitoring their weight and policing their appetites while pathologizing those who go too far. Finally, by highlighting the continuity between the mentality of Pro-Anas and the everyday thoughts and behaviors of "normal" women who dislike their bodies, a continuum suggests that dieting is a doorway that can lead to more dangerous eating patterns.

The supporters of Ana view anorexia as a religion, or something very akin to it. This is disturbing—and yet perhaps not all that unexpected if we consider the quasi-religious aspects of today's popular pursuit of slenderness, with its mythical, symbolic, sacrificial, ritualizing, ascetic, penitential, dogmatic, and devotional dimensions. Indeed, for many women—not just the Pro-Anas—the never-ending quest for a fat-free body *has* come to function like a religion.

Unlike Pro-Anas, though, most of us do not describe the drama of our food and body struggles in explicitly religious terms. Yet the spiritual urges masked by eating problems lurk just beneath the surface of our compulsive thinking and behavior. Many women describe a deep emptiness—an insatiable hunger—that bingeing, restricting, dieting, excessive exercising and a host of other dysfunctional behaviors related to eating and body image aim to fill.

How much mental energy have you devoted to wishing your stomach was flatter or your thighs thinner? How many days have you filled counting calories? How many hours have you spent in the gym? How much of your life has been preoccupied with binging, purging, and starving yourself?

With so much of our energy consumed by the all-encompassing fantasy of thinness, it's hard to remember the goals and visions we once held dear. With so much of our time preoccupied with the goal of losing weight, other pursuits get put on hold. By adopting the idea that thinness equals happiness, some of us even become willing to sacrifice anything in pursuit of the perfect body. Author Pamela Houston reflects:

> For a good part of my life, I would have quite literally given anything to be thin . . . a finger, three toes, the sight of one eye . . . For the majority of my lifetime I would have traded being ugly, deformed, and thin for being pretty, whole, and fat.[6]

Feelings of emptiness, yearning, pain, and release expose the passion—a strange mixture of suffering and desire—that permeates our troubled relationships with our bodies. If passion is a spiritual energy that seeks harmony, freedom, and interconnection, then I believe that a preoccupation with weight and eating, no matter how minor or severe, reveals a passion that has not yet found an adequate outlet. You may be hungry for a way to feel empowered in a society that seems out of control, create meaning in a world that seems meaningless, or resolve feelings of depression, restlessness, or anxiety. You may be looking for a path—an ultimate purpose.

I would characterize these "hungers" as spiritual. We need to discover our true purpose in life. We need meaningful symbols, beliefs, and stories by which to organize our day-to-day lives and derive meaning from our existence. We need a way to understand our universe and our place in it, to see things from a "bigger perspective," and to experience ourselves as fully alive.

Traditionally these needs have been filled by religion. While Christianity has been dominant in the West, people all over the world have found and created meaning through a wide variety of faiths. However, traditional religion no longer plays a central role in the lives of increasing numbers of women. Yet their spiritual needs have not diminished. In fact, in the face of our contemporary society, where established values have been largely overshadowed by a commercially-driven, consumer-oriented culture, these spiritual hungers have grown to mammoth proportions. Even for those women who have stayed connected to organized religion, the often patriarchal and fundamentalist character of some forms of worship may may not nourish their deepest spiritual needs and desires.

In the absence of other, more fulfilling means to satisfy these spiritual hungers, the masses have turned to what I call "The Religion of Thinness." Like those extremists who worship Ana, they have become devoted to the idols and images that provide us with an ideal of female beauty. They have used rituals like counting calories or binging and purging to feel safe and pure. They have embraced the symbols and stories of weight loss as a method for generating life's meaning and have adopted a distinctly *religious* attitude toward the quest for thinness and the perfect body. This has become their daily path and ultimate purpose.

Religion: The Role It Plays and What Happens When It's Lost

Religion is rooted in our need and search for meaning and fulfillment. One vital difference between us and other living creatures is our quest to understand the purpose of our existence and to experience wellness and accomplishment in relation to that purpose. We want to know what our lives are about and how we should live, and we long to experience ourselves as healthy and satisfied. In various times, circumstances, and places, people have turned to religions to guide them on this journey toward insight and well-being.

Expressions of religious devotion are richly varied. Consider the ecstatic dances of indigenous shamans with healing powers, the prostrations and prayers that Muslims perform in honor of and submission to God ("Allah" in Arabic), the cross-legged, straight-postured meditation of Buddhists who focus their energies on simply breathing, the lighting of candles by Jewish women to welcome the Sabbath at the end of the week, the crowds of Hindus ritually bathing in the Ganges, or the heartfelt hymns of Christians congregated in churches, singing praise and thanksgiving to their beloved Savior. Despite such diversity, all religions share the goal of connecting people to a greater power than themselves, a reality that lies both beyond and within the world we comprehend with our physical senses.

The varied relationships we have to established religions are due in part to their ambiguous nature. The word *religion* is derived from a Latin verb that means "to bind," which can have either a connecting or restricting effect. Religion has functioned in both ways throughout human history, fostering animosity and hatred as well as selflessness and peace. In the words of Swami Vivekananda, "No other human interest has deluged the world in so much blood as religion; at the same time nothing has built so many hospitals and asylums for the poor… as religion. Nothing makes us so cruel as religion, nothing makes us so tender."[7] As an instrument for cultivating our search for meaning, religion can be a resource for empowerment and integration. But, it can also be a tool of oppression, reinforcing obedience to external authority and restricting us to a closed or narrow point of view.

Religious Oppression and Its Role in Supporting The Religion of Thinness

In recent decades, the oppressive potential of religion has been called into question, and it is largely because of this quality that the authority of established traditions has been somewhat shaken. One group that has been particularly affected by religious oppression is women. To varying degrees, all the major world religions contain beliefs, symbols, texts, and rituals that are patriarchal. Christianity has numerous examples. Christian misogyny is epitomized by the words of the 3rd century Church Father, Tertullian, who depicted women as "the devil's gateway," along with numerous other theologians' references to women as spiritually "inferior" or "weak."

If you identify as a Christian, you may or may not have considered some of the more patriarchal aspects of this tradition. Nonetheless, the oppression of women in Christianity isn't restricted to men like Tertullian. Biblical stories from Genesis onward have been given misogynistic readings for centuries. It was Eve who ate the forbidden fruit and caused humanity to fall into sin. God is invariably envisioned as a man, and even the Holy Spirit, originally described in Hebrew as a feminine noun (*ruach*), became neuter in Greek (*pneuma*), and eventually masculine in Latin (*spiritus*). Although Mary, the mother of Christ, holds a special place in Christianity (most prominently in Catholicism), her sexuality has been stripped from her by her status as a "virgin." At the opposite extreme from Christ's virgin mother is another Mary—Mary Magdalene—who was given the reputation of being a whore (despite the lack of historical evidence supporting this view) and therefore needed Christ to save her. And although the New Testament attests to Mary Magdalene as one of Jesus' most faithful followers—she remains at the foot of the cross when most of the male disciples flee in fear, and all four gospels identify her as the first to witness the empty tomb—the memory of her has been both tainted and obscured by male interpreters.

It's interesting to note that each of these examples involves the physical body of women. According to the Genesis myth, sin entered the world through the disobedient appetite of a woman—Eve ate the forbidden fruit. She was the devil's gateway. Christ was only able to enter the world through the "pure," desexualized body of a virgin. And even without supporting evidence, Mary Magdalene gained the reputation for having an unruly sexuality, her primary sin.

However, Christianity is not the only religion guilty of patriarchy, misogyny, and female oppression. Examples from other traditions abound. In some denominations of Judaism, men recite a daily prayer to thank God for not having been born a woman, slave, or gentile. While Muslim women are said to have equal standing before God, they have little opportunity for leadership in their mosques. One sacred Hindu text suggests that the "female principle" tends to be evil and dangerous if unaccompanied by the "male principle." And in Buddhism, some older sects argue that being born female is the negative consequence of karma from a past life.[8]

Throughout this book I critique some of the patriarchal aspects of these religious traditions. I do so, not because I believe that any of them are intrinsically bad or wrong and therefore incapable of nourishing women spiritually, but because their misogynistic tendencies leave women vulnerable to the false promises of The Religion of Thinness.

You will find that I am particularly critical of Christianity. Given the patriarchal leanings in each of the traditions just mentioned (and many others not named), you may wonder why I am so hard on this faith in particular. The truth is that I am not necessarily more critical of Christianity than other religions in this regard. I think that all traditions with a history of oppressing women should be closely scrutinized. However, I *do* put Christianity under a microscope, and I do so for important reasons.

First, no other religion has had as much influence on Western culture as Christianity. Christian ideas and institutions have enjoyed a dominant position in the West for over 16 centuries. The result is that we are all influenced either directly or indirectly by its traditions, ideas, and beliefs—whether or not we are Christian.

Second, and perhaps even more important in the context of this book, Christianity has a long legacy of fostering associations between women, sin, and bodily cravings (note the examples just given). At the same time, it has promised women (either implicitly or explicitly) that salvation lies in the mastery of these appetites and in their subordination to a higher (male) power. These constructs are complicit with The Religion of Thinness and have been used over and over to support it in some rather blatant ways, including, but certainly not limited to, the Christian diet movement that you will learn more about in Chapter 5.

Of course, many women continue to find meaning and support from traditional religions, despite their male biases. This is not because they are ignorant or duped. On the contrary, these women recognize that they *do* indeed have spiritual needs and many intentionally draw on the resources of their religions that are most spiritually nourishing to them. They may also reinterpret symbols and beliefs in ways that speak to and support their own experience.

In fact, a growing number of feminist Christians are developing new readings of their tradition that empower women and establish the critical role they have played in its history. These readings highlight how Jesus challenged the social conventions of his time and treated all people as equals, how women like Mary Magdalene played a crucial role in the early Christian movement, and how Jesus' vision of holiness was not based on body-denying disciplines but is best captured in the image of a festive banquet to which *everyone*—tax collectors, prostitutes, the poor, women, and all the other "unholy" people—was invited.[9] Feminist theologians continue to uncover historical examples of Christian women whose faith was a source of strength and intelligence. When a group of male ministers ordered the 19th century Black abolitionist Sojourner Truth to sit down and be quiet because women were not supposed to speak in public (thanks to the sin of Eve), Truth quickly responded that if the first woman was strong enough to turn the whole world upside down, then that just proved the power of women to change the world—and, she informed them, that's what she was going to do!

Regardless of our relationship to institutionalized faith, most of us long for a way to make sense of the puzzles and pains of our lives. We need rituals for celebrating life's joys and transitions, and we need resources for channeling our creativity and passion. These needs do not wither away when traditional religions fail to adequately nourish them. Instead, they drive us to look for other ways to feed our hungry spirits.

Ways like The Religion of Thinness.

Filling the Void with The Religion of Thinness

Our crusade to be thinner masks a greater hunger for a life that is meaningful and fulfilling. Historically, religions have provided the primary resources for addressing this yearning. Jews, Christians, and Muslims refer to the wholeness we seek as salvation. Hindus speak of *moksha*, and Buddhists of enlightenment. You may connect with some of these traditional concepts or you may not. In any case, for many of us today, including those who consider themselves "religious," traditional faith no longer functions as the primary resource for finding fulfillment and coping with the difficulties of our lives.

Alongside traditional religion, a plethora of non-religious alternatives offer solutions to what were once considered issues of the soul. Psychotherapy (literally "soul healing"), self-help books, seminars, and the like provide guidance and tools for people seeking healing and wholeness in their lives. In addition, a growing number of Westerners have turned to new age alternatives and traditions from the East, going to ashrams, practicing yoga, or trying various meditation techniques. In different ways, these alternatives offer solutions to those who don't wish to couch their pursuit of well-being in conventional religious terms, or those who do wish to supplement their traditional faith with other tools for spiritual growth.

Amidst these options has risen The Religion of Thinness—a secular faith with a loosely organized set of rituals, symbols, stories, images, and beliefs that:

1. Gives us what some theologians refer to as an *ultimate concern*, or (what I call) an *ultimate purpose*. This concept was developed by the 20th century Protestant theologian, Paul Tillich. For him, it meant God. But he points out that many people adopt an ultimate concern that isn't ultimate at all. Instead, their choice reflects a sense of purpose that is shaped by social norms, self-interested desires, etc. This can be thought of as an ultimate purpose, or the fundamental underlying reasons you are alive, including your deepest values, your most cherished ideals, the real goals of your life, etc. In the case of The Religion of Thinness, the ultimate purpose is thinness, which clearly isn't ultimate in the grand scheme of things, but we nonetheless embrace it as our most precious ideal.

2. Gives us a set of myths to believe in regarding the rewards of thinness. Every day we are inundated with tales about the wonderful lives thin people lead. With stories, images, headlines, and a number of other tactics, the media convinces us that if we, too, can "perfect" our bodies, our lives will be "perfected" in turn. This myth gives us something to believe in, some hope to hang on to, despite the fact that the promise it offers is empty.

3. Presents us with iconographic imagery to which we can aspire. We are saturated by images of flawless female bodies daily, and most of us desperately wish to live up to those ideals. These images are akin to religious iconography. They inspire us and offer us hope through achieving that "beautiful" slender body.

4. Offers rituals by which to organize our daily lives. Counting calories, monitoring what we eat, checking our weight on the scale, exercising compulsively, starving, binging, purging—all become ritualized for many women who are preoccupied with the pursuit of thinness. Whereas anorexic rituals focus on restriction, bulimics cycle through relinquishing control only to regain and eventually lose it again. Those who eat compulsively usually do so in predetermined ways (at certain times of day, in front of the TV, with their favorite "binge foods," etc.).

5. Creates a set of moral rules and vocabulary by which we can judge ourselves and others. Diet plans are particularly rife with language regarding "good" foods and "bad" foods. It's likely you have adopted some of this language and the thinking it promotes. Are you "bad" if you eat dessert? Are you "good" if you don't? Do you judge your self-worth by the number on the scale? These are all moral judgments.

6. Includes us in a community of women who are all trying to achieve the same objectives. Through weight loss rituals and the mythology they support, we are connected to other women who share our longing for a slender body. How many of your conversations revolve around weight loss? Women rely on such discussions to bond with each other. Why do you think commercial weight-loss programs are so popular? When we join, we become a member of a community. In an age when communities are evaporating, the shared pursuit of a slender body gives us a way to feel connected.

7. Promises salvation. The ultimate promise of The Religion of Thinness is nothing short of salvation. We are told that by achieving the perfect body we will achieve the health, happiness, and well-being we've been looking for. And we believe that our problems will fall away with the pounds we shed.

Note that each of these aspects of The Religion of Thinness (i.e., ultimate purpose, myths, icons, rituals, morals, community, and salvation) was historically accounted for by traditional religion in order to address specific spiritual needs. These are the resources by which religion helps us create meaning in our lives and connect both to the people around us and to something larger than ourselves. These needs are at the very core of human existence, and when we don't have adequate means to address them, we will likely look for substitutes to feed our hungry spirits. Looking back on her journey into anorexia, one young woman reflected: "Dieting eventually became a replacement religion for me, with its own set of commandments and rituals. I was so devoted that I was practically ready to give up my life for it."[10]

Why So Many Women Embrace The Religion of Thinness

Despite the increase in male eating disorders and men's growing preoccupation with both thinness and muscularity, there is a clear gender imbalance in The Religion of Thinness that leans toward women. This imbalance stems from both the shifting social roles of men and women in the latter half of the 20th century and the double standards that still linger, despite these changes.

Historically, men have been encouraged to find meaning in life by developing their minds, whereas women have been taught to rely upon their appearance. Men are supposed to be *attracted* (to women); therefore, women are advised to make themselves sexually *attractive* (to men). Men are urged to pursue their dreams and satisfy their cravings, while women learn to sacrifice their own needs for the sake of others. Men's concerns have been institutionalized, whereas women's have been routinely trivialized. These outdated social standards are, unfortunately, still very powerful today.

The prevalence of these double standards explains why the majority of those who are drawn to The Religion of Thinness are women. Consciously or not, this secular faith helps them achieve many of our culture's conventional notions of what it means to be a woman by:

- helping them become more "attractive"

- rewarding them for focusing their energies on their appearance rather than developing their intelligence and creativity

- encouraging them to sacrifice their own pleasure by denying their hunger for the sake of winning the approval of others

- magnifying the importance of something as petty as the size of their bodies and diverting their attention away from their real needs and concerns

- giving them jurisdiction over the two areas of life that have traditionally been assigned to women—food and their bodies

Curiously, women's faith in thinness gained momentum during the decades (late 1960s–1980s) when the feminist movement was making strides to unleash their intellectual and creative powers. Therapist Kim Chernin believes this timing is not coincidental and that the increased pressure on women to be thin was, in part, a cultural backlash to the expansion of women's consciousness. She notes the strikingly different language between feminist groups of this era and those who were devoted to weight loss. In the feminist sphere, women sought to *acquire* weight, to *gain* greater power and gravity, to *enlarge* or widen their frame of influence, to *expand* and *develop* their passions. Meanwhile, the dieting groups that emerged during that period encouraged women to make themselves *smaller*, to *reduce* their impact, to be-*little* themselves, to *restrict* their appetites and *control* their yearnings.[11]

Even women who seem otherwise liberated find themselves enslaved by the fantasy of thinness. The widespread attraction of this fantasy reveals just how deeply entrenched the fear of female flesh and appetite remains in this culture. Despite the successes of the feminist movement, many of us still unconsciously adopt narrow, chauvinistic ideas about what it means to *be* a woman. For those born and raised in a culture that worships female slenderness, these outdated notions are not easily overcome.

Somewhere deep inside, you know that to be a whole person you don't have to be thin. But do you truly hear that voice? Are you able to believe it? Can you live by its wisdom instead of the images and ideals of The Religion of Thinness? If you are a devotee as I once was, you are probably having a hard time doing that. Even when you know intellectually that the promises of The Religion of Thinness are empty, accepting this truth and finding new ways of creating meaning is a real challenge.

I've found that in order to break habitual patterns of thoughts and behaviors about food and our bodies, we must understand how The Religion of Thinness functions in our lives. We need to learn how to become critical of the messages we receive that serve to support its oppressive, misogynistic, bigoted, and controlling nature. And we have to be alert to the underlying spiritual dynamics of our misbegotten desire to be thin and find more nourishing ways to feed our hungry spirits.

The Spiritual Dynamics of Eating Problems

Many people equate spirituality with religion, and though they are often connected, they are actually quite distinct. Religions are organized systems of symbols, rituals, myths, and beliefs. They tend to be institutionalized and provide a worldview for a community of believers. Spirituality has more of an experiential quality. It is the *inner* dimension of religious life—the process through which many of us create and discover the meaning of our lives. It grounds and connects our life experiences and encompasses and permeates our everyday disappointments and dreams, anxieties, and longings. It is a practice, a path, a discipline. It is how we connect to that which we hold sacred.[12] Spirituality puts us in touch with the creative and transformative energy propelling us from one day to another, from one moment to the next.

When our spirituality is dormant, our lives often feel empty. You may actually be unaware that your spirit is hungry, because judging and controlling your body distances you from your feelings, thoughts, desires, and needs. And so, unconsciously, you search for *something* to help you feel alive again. Maybe that something is the physical feeling of hunger. Perhaps it is the sensation of eating, an act that brings our minds and bodies together, just as starving ourselves seems to drive them apart. It could be the fantasy of thinness, which always gives us something to strive for, something to look forward to, the happy ending. In any case, based on the amount of time and energy we spend worrying about how to look and what, how much, and whether or not to eat, it's clear that, for many of us, our spiritual needs have been engulfed by an enormous black hole—one that we unconsciously hope to fill with the The Religion of Thinness.

You may be unable to recognize your spiritual needs for a variety of reasons. People for whom religion was not a significant part of their upbringing or who have lost faith may not think of themselves as religious and may assume they don't *have* spiritual needs. Those who *do* consider themselves religious often have narrow ideas about what spiritual needs are. A woman who struggled with compulsive eating asked her therapist in exasperation: "I go to church, say my prayers, and read the Bible everyday. So why do I still feel this vacuum inside my soul?"

Tragically, The Religion of Thinness shortchanges our hungry spirits, ultimately deepening the emptiness it promises to fill. Much of what this pseudo-faith offers is the spiritual equivalent of junk food: the glossy images of models who function as icons of feminine perfection, the exercise rituals that promise renewed life in the form of firmer buttocks, and the belief that health, beauty, and happiness depend on the shape of our bodies. No wonder a part of us feels so malnourished! Those of us who have fallen into this superficial scheme of salvation have done so not because of a lack of intelligence, but because we have not learned to identify—much less adequately address—our genuine needs.

Exploring the spiritual dimension of your life may bring these needs to the surface. Is it possible that what you really want is beyond the yearning to be thin? Perhaps, beneath your great efforts to erase your body and contain its cravings, there is a desire to connect with your flesh, to be at home in your own skin, to experience the power of life that animates your body and enlivens your spirit. For the more we get in touch with the needs of our hearts and souls, the more our faith in thinness loses its importance.

Spirituality as an Alternative to
The Religion of Thinness

There is a story of a wise teacher, who was asked by a struggling student for a metaphor to explain the elusive nature of spirituality. Staring at a massive stone fireplace in the room where the two women were seated, the teacher pondered the request. Finally, with her eyes fixed on the mortar that held the many stones together, she explained, "Spirituality is not something you can isolate from everything else. It's not one particular stone in the fireplace that you can distinguish from the others. Rather, like the mortar, spirituality is that which holds the stones together, connecting all of them to one another."[13]

When we feel spiritually disconnected, we spend a great deal of time and energy trying to do whatever we can to "keep it all together." In a world that strips us of the time we truly need to do our work well, take care of ourselves, be present to our families and friends, and be creative, we *do* often feel like things are falling apart. For some women, monitoring what and how much they eat or exercise seems to give them a way of regaining control over their lives.

But when we are spiritually well-nourished, we trust the power of life that sustains us and holds the disparate stones of our lives in place, allowing us to let go and connect with what really matters. Spirituality frees us from the endless and futile attempts to keep our lives in neat and tidy order by attempting to keep our bodies flawless and slim. It fosters the wisdom to accept and the strength to deal with whatever challenges come our way. In this sense, it is both an antidote and an alternative to The Religion of Thinness.

In their groundbreaking work, *Spiritual Approaches in the Treatment of Women with Eating Disorders*, P. Scott Richards, Randy K. Hardman, and Michael E. Berrett explore the role of spirituality in the treatment and recovery process. They were motivated to write this book because their patients repeatedly told them that their faith was one of the most powerful catalysts for positive change. They cite numerous research studies indicating that spiritual beliefs and practices play an important, if not central, role in recovery. The concluding chapter features messages from recovering patients to other women with eating disorders about the importance of faith and spirituality. Some of the insights and suggestions they offer include:

> "God is like a gentle mother who sang the world into creation and holds each one of us as a precious baby."

> "Spiritual growth is more empowering, long-lasting, and comforting than the eating disorder ever was or ever will be."

> "Be brave! Gaining your faith back and accepting God's love is immensely hard, but it is worth it in the end."

> "Count your blessings. Look for the good things, and be grateful for each and every thing in your life. . ."[14]

These encouraging words underscore the pivotal role spirituality plays in the healing process. Remembering what matters most in life empowers us to do the inner work necessary for recovering our bodies and spirits. Reconnecting with what we hold sacred allows our struggling spirits to rest. In contrast to The Religion of Thinness, which traps us inside our individual egos by gluing our attention to the size and shape of our bodies, spirituality connects us to all of life in its infinite manifestations, including those parts of the world and ourselves that make us uncomfortable or afraid. It enables us to embrace the *fullness* of life as it actually is—with all its ups and downs.

Spirituality provides the courage to face our problems and embrace our passions by linking us to a power that is both within and greater than ourselves: a power that is already holding everything together, even when we feel like things might come apart. Strengthening our relationship with this greater power—regardless of what we call it— enables us to stop trying so hard to play God with our lives. Spirituality gives us the courage to let go of our need to have things be a certain way. It allows us to touch that vulnerable place inside: the place that is inherently unstable, uncertain, unfinished, and unsatisfied.

This is the place of opportunity, as spiritual author Pema Chödrön writes, "We can let the circumstances of our lives harden us and make us increasingly resentful and afraid, or we can let them soften us and make us kinder."[15] The problem with The Religion of Thinness is that in the process of tightening our bodies it simultaneously hardens our hearts. The underlying quest for control is essentially at odds with authentic faith, which involves openness and trust, not conquest and certainty. By relying on such strategies as denial, fantasy, restraint, escape, and judgment to deal with the challenges of our lives, The Religion of Thinness prevents us from cultivating the genuine bravery we need to transform these challenges into inner wisdom.

Practicing Peace with Our Bodies by Becoming Mindful

Where does such bravery come from? How can you find the strength you need to extricate yourself from The Religion of Thinness?

Such courage develops with practice. It grows out of our repeated efforts—despite setbacks—to change how we think about food and how we live in our bodies. We cannot wait until we feel spiritually strong enough to begin this journey. We become spiritually strong by opening to new situations and feelings, letting go when we want control, and remembering what truly matters. Ultimately, the courage we need to release our obsession emerges as we practice being present to the very feelings that our eating and body image problems have enabled us to avoid.

So much of our suffering stems from our resistance to "what is." We refuse to accept our bodies as they are. We treat our hunger like an alien intruder. We berate ourselves for feeling depressed or anxious and either eat or starve to avoid emotions and situations that scare us. Our general attitude is often, "This is not how it's supposed to be!"

If, instead of fighting what is, we could cultivate an attitude of acceptance, the suffering that comes from wanting things to be different would be greatly diminished.

Accepting your body requires getting in touch with the thoughts, feelings, and bodily sensations you experience without judging or becoming attached to them. It means fully feeling the curves and bulges, the muscle and fat, as well as the life energy inside you, and experiencing your feelings about your body and appearance without becoming enveloped in them. You must move into the position of the "observer self" and "watch" your physical, psychological, and spiritual experiences.

Doing this requires that you get in touch with what you are experiencing right now, this very moment. You must learn to slow down enough to be aware of your thoughts, feelings, and sensations to tap into that part of you that transcends the ideas you have about your weight and body.

Getting and staying present to our inner experience is how we *practice peace with our bodies*, a phrase developed by eating disorder therapist Cissy Brady-Rogers to describe the process of healing. Practicing peace with our bodies means learning to fully inhabit, care for, appreciate, and enjoy the very flesh we have patrolled, feared, loathed, and punished. As the Buddhist monk Thich Nhat Hanh reminds us, practicing peace need not be elaborate or esoteric, and we don't need to go elsewhere to get started:

> Peace is present right here and now, in ourselves and in everything we do and see. The question is whether or not we are in touch with it. We don't have to travel far away to enjoy the blue sky. We don't have to leave our city or even our neighborhood to enjoy the eyes of a beautiful child. Even the air we breathe can be a source of joy. We can smile, breathe, walk, and eat our meals in a way that allows us to be in touch with the abundance of happiness that is available.[16]

The key to experiencing such peace is the ability to be fully present to our lives, which depends on being present in our bodies without judging them (something most adherents to The Religion of Thinness find it difficult to do). We develop this ability through the practice of *mindfulness*.

Mindfulness is a spiritual discipline that is rooted in Eastern meditation traditions. It is also closely related to other spiritual practices, perhaps most notably the common practice of prayer. What connects these different spiritual techniques for cultivating peace is their emphasis on *paying attention*. Mindfulness is a way of being and thinking in which one becomes fully immersed in the present moment. And when we are fully present in the now, virtually anything we do can become a prayer. As the Methodist scholar of religion Diana Eck notes, prayer is simply "attention of the heart."[17] Mindfulness focuses on the quality of our experience rather than a specific belief or dogma. Thus it is a technique for cultivating peace that people can apply regardless of their spiritual background. It gives us a way to challenge The Religion of Thinness by waking us up to its false promises while nourishing the spiritual needs that drew us to it.[18]

We practice mindfulness by doing what we are doing without concern for the past or the future. There are countless ways to do this, such as:

- Eating a quiet meal without distractions like reading, talking, watching TV, listening to music, or working at the computer

- Experiencing the tingling refreshment of your skin when you bathe

- Being witness to the multiple ways your organs function without any conscious effort or attention on your part— your heart, lungs, and brain, for instance

- Paying attention to the strength of your legs as they carry you up the stairs

- Enjoying a hot cup of tea, taking time to sip it slowly and feel the warmth it brings to your body

Mindfulness focuses your undivided attention on the activity at hand. By immersing yourself in the present moment, mindfulness liberates you from the anxieties of and rules around food that preoccupy your psyche: *What will I eat (or not eat) tonight for dinner? How many calories were in that muffin? How many more miles to go on the treadmill?*

Do these jeans make me look fat? When thoughts like these arise, practicing mindfulness interrupts their flow and makes you aware of how often you are preoccupied with food and your body.

As you learn to watch such mental meanderings without judging, indulging, or denying them, you also become aware of the reality that *you are not your negative thoughts.* In doing so, you return to your body as it is in the present, where you can experience the peace that is already within you.

Mindfulness is one of the primary tools this book offers for deconstructing The Religion of Thinness. In every chapter, I teach mindfulness techniques that come from a variety of sources and span different religious, spiritual, and psychotherapeutic traditions. However, the key point to each of them is always the same—giving up your resistance to *what is* by becoming aware of your experience, right *here*, right *now*, in *this* moment.

Although mindfulness is a serious spiritual practice, we don't need to become somber or pious about it. Becoming mindful enables us to appreciate and take pleasure in our lives. Even the most scrumptious piece of chocolate won't be very satisfying if we are not consciously aware of how it tastes. Yet a bowl of plain brown rice can be astonishingly delicious if we eat it slowly and deliberately. Ultimately, our capacity to enjoy both the "chocolate" *and* the "rice" of our lives depends on our ability to be present to them.

To begin experiencing the power of the present moment through mindfulness, try the following technique. It is one of the cornerstones of mindfulness practice, and I mention it throughout this book.

Sitting Still and Watching Your Breath

Sitting still and watching your breath is a classic mindfulness technique. Though often thought of as meditation, it is perhaps more accurately described as "just sitting." You don't meditate on an idea. You don't force your thoughts in any particular direction. You just sit quietly and notice any thoughts, feelings, and/or bodily sensations that come up, without attaching to them or judging them. This practice can be enhanced by paying attention to (and sometimes counting) your breath as it naturally comes in and goes out of your body without any effort on the part of your conscious mind.

You don't need special cushions or esoteric postures. All you really need is the willingness to slow down, be still, pay attention to your breathing, and see what happens inside you. Even five minutes a few times a week can be helpful, especially if you are just beginning. I recommend you start with shorter sessions and gradually build up. It may take a while for your mind to settle down from its typical, rambunctious habits, but the more often you do it, the easier it will be. Regularly carving time out of your days to practice will keep you more consistent and will help develop your capacity to observe your thoughts, be present in your body, and be aware of the present moment.

Below are a few key suggestions for sitting and watching your breath. Use them to bring yourself back to the present moment when you feel drawn into obsessive thinking or behavior, or as a starting point for some of the other exercises in the book.

1. Find a comfortable, quiet place to sit. Sitting and watching your breath is about accepting your experience—whatever it is—and not about seeking quiet or comfort. However, as you begin practicing, it is easy to get distracted and drawn into your thoughts or the activities around you. Sitting in a room where kids are running around screaming and bouncing off the walls isn't going to be conducive to experiencing the present moment! So find a quiet place where you won't be disturbed. I recommend gently closing your eyes to become more centered, but you can also leave them open.

2. Keep your back straight. Whether you sit on a cushion on the floor or a chair, good posture will help you remain attentive and make it easier to focus on the air moving through your torso. Shunryu Suzuki Roshi says in his book *Zen Mind, Beginner's Mind* that "the posture is the practice" because if you lose your posture, you lose the state of alertness that observing your thoughts requires. It also facilitates proper breathing, which will help draw you into the present by keeping your attention relaxed but watchful.

3. Breathe from your belly. Most of us don't know how to breathe. In fact, if you are preoccupied with your body and, in particular, the size of your stomach, you may resist properly expanding it. Deep breathing originates in your diaphragm as it naturally expands and contracts, without any commands from your conscious mind. This expansion and contraction is what draws air in and pushes it out of your lungs. That means when you breathe deeply and naturally, you breathe with your belly, not with your chest.

Try placing one hand over your heart and one hand on your belly. If the hand on your belly rises and falls with your breath, you are breathing properly. If the hand on your chest rises and falls, you are still breathing with your chest and need to retrain your breathing. Continue making an effort to breathe from your belly as you observe your internal experience and stay present.

4. Watch and/or count your breath. What does it mean to "watch your breath"? Of course you can't do this literally. I'm referring to the act of consciously bringing attention to your breathing. Simply watching your breath can interrupt the stream of compulsive thinking by returning you to the present, since you are breathing *right now.*

One way to tune in is to count your breaths. As you sit, try counting each exhalation from one to 10, and then start over again. If you lose track because your mind is distracted by a thought, that's okay. Again, without judging yourself, simply bring your awareness back to your breath and resume counting.

5. Sit still. Try not to move around too much as you sit. Pain may come up, especially if you sit cross-legged. So may boredom, loneliness, fear, craving, agitation, fatigue, and many other sensations. Don't move to escape these experiences. Instead, sink into the present moment and notice what is going on for you without judging it, without trying to get rid of it, without running from it. Simply remain still and watchful. If you are in pain and you *must* move, adjust your position and then resume stillness.

Stilling your body allows you the opportunity to witness the busyness of your mind—all the thinking, feeling, and planning that draw you out of the present moment. Observing this process as it's happening, rather than being completely lost in it, is a moment of awakening and an important step in loosening the grip of your obsession and embracing a deeper sense of who you are.

6. Watch your thoughts, feelings, and bodily sensations as they arise, without attaching to them. As was just mentioned, stilling your body doesn't necessarily still your mind. A myriad of thoughts and feelings will continue to drift into your awareness while you practice sitting and breathing, but let them pass like fallen leaves being carried away by a river's current. Mindfulness entails watching the leaves of our mind float by instead of holding onto them, examining their details, or judging them.

Although this practice is relatively simple, it can be a challenge. You may have to bring yourself back to the present moment 100 times in the course of five minutes! But this is absolutely fine—you are learning a new skill. Sitting is about practice, not perfection.

The experience of consciously sitting and breathing reflects the connection between breath and spirit that is found in some languages. In Latin, for example, the root for *spirit* means *breathe*, and the one for *inspire* is *breathe into*. In Hebrew, the word for spirit is *ruach*, which literally means *breath* or *wind*. This noun is used in the opening chapter of the Bible to speak of the maternal, life-giving Spirit that hovered and ruminated over the abyss at the dawn of Creation. In the following chapter, which recounts the story about the Garden of Eden, the Spirit that enlivens all of nature is breathed into Adam and Eve, who represent the first human beings, suggesting that all people are filled with the Spirit-given breath of life.[19]

The link between the life that is both beyond and within us suggests that our spirit is not a ghost imprisoned inside our body. It is a dimension of ourselves—our consciousness, energy, and presence—that emanates from and is grounded in our bodies and connects us to the surrounding flow of life. Though we experience ourselves through our individual human form, our spirit is part of a *larger* spirit—the "Life of life" as the Benedictine sister Joan Chittister calls it[21]—that permeates all of Creation. When we feel the presence of this life-giving spirit within ourselves, we experience an inner calm and peace, regardless of our size or shape.

Whatever our religious background or beliefs, when we find ourselves stressing about weight and eating, we can practice mindfulness by returning our awareness to our breath, coming into our bodies, and reconnecting with the miraculous power of life that simultaneously transcends and flows through us. This practice can also be used to relieve stress or deal with difficult thoughts or emotions, and it can be especially useful when you find yourself obsessing about food and thinness.

Learning to Be a Cultural Critic

In addition to mindfulness, the other tool I want to offer you for dismantling The Religion of Thinness is cultural criticism. As we will see, these practices are connected. But whereas mindfulness increases our awareness by focusing attention on our inner experience, cultural criticism shifts that attention to our external environment and helps us recognize and evaluate the messages we are constantly imbibing on an unconscious level. Unlike mindfulness practice, cultural criticism requires us to use our analytical mind, to examine and reflect on the storylines that surround us so that we can understand their impact within us.

Cultural criticism of The Religion of Thinness begins with a crucial insight: *women are not born believing that they should be thin*. Rather, they are indoctrinated into this belief by a society that glorifies the slender ideal. Despite its obvious social foundation, however, faith in the saving grace of thinness is often experienced as a private revelation. Feeding our need for a sense of purpose, losing weight feels like an individual achievement, while gaining weight feels like a personal failure. This is because most of us have *internalized* our culture's mandate for slenderness, incorporating it into our everyday thoughts and feelings and making it our own.

However, by identifying the societal influences that encourage our seemingly personal preoccupations with food and body image, we can learn to transform our thinking. From this perspective, our problems with food are not the result of our lack of will-power; they are the product of a culture that thrives on our feelings of shame and body-hatred. We are *conditioned* to believe there's something wrong with our bodies, and certain industries capitalize on that feeling. It's no wonder we feel so alienated from our bodies. The more aware we become of how we've internalized this value of thinness, the freer we will be to stop judging ourselves and change the thought patterns and behaviors that get us stuck. A recovering anorexic-bulimic woman explained:

> I used to blame myself for my eating disorder. I thought it was a reflection of my own weakness. Now, I understand that I didn't bring my illness on by myself. I had plenty of help from the magazines I read and even from my friends who were always talking about needing to lose weight. I wanted very badly to be *someone* in the eyes of the world, and everything seemed to tell me that being noticeably skinny was the best way to do this.

Becoming critical of the societal forces that manufacture and drive our faith in thinness is an integral part of the paradigm shift that moves us out of The Religion of Thinness. When we scrutinize the dominant views of our culture—media images, medical studies, government reports, moral authorities—instead of criticizing our bodies, we are practicing *cultural criticism*. This involves questioning our assumptions and challenging the social norms and ideals we have unknowingly taken for granted. But critical thinking is not just an academic exercise. It is also a spiritual practice because it is about transforming our consciousness so we can be more awake to ourselves and to the world we live in.

Cultural Criticism as a Spiritual Practice

All great spiritual leaders advocated and practiced cultural criticism. The ancient Hebrew prophets cried out against prevailing injustices committed against the poor by those who idolized money and power. Following in their footsteps, Jesus of Nazareth denounced the dominant social and religious stipulations that put laws above human well-being.

The revelations received by the prophet Muhammad defied a society rife with class divisions by insisting that all persons are equal in the eyes of God. Similarly, The Buddha challenged the status quo by condemning the caste system and by providing a path to enlightenment that *all* people could follow. Mahatma Gandhi's religious convictions led him to wage a successful non-violent battle against British imperialism. Drawing on the teachings of both Jesus and Gandhi, the peaceful defiance of Dr. Martin Luther King, Jr., helped transform a society stratified by racial divisions. Indeed, there are numerous examples of visionary leaders throughout history whose ideals are rooted in countercultural values that challenge traditional myths and assumptions.

In various ways, the lives and teachings of these leaders illustrate the power of a culturally-aware perspective. Each of them challenged their contemporaries to replace blind faith with *critical consciousness* by examining the real sources of human suffering and alienation. Each questioned the "false gods" of their time—the idolatries of wealth, legalism, power, racial dominance—encouraging others to protest social injustice. Each pointed to a greater vision of wholeness, a different kind of ideal, and an alternative way of seeing and being.

Cultural criticism is a basic tool and a foundational practice used throughout this book to challenge various aspects of The Religion of Thinness. Developing this skill can help you experience your inherent wisdom—that inner place of clarity and insight that knows when something is or isn't right, when to say "yes" and when to say "no," what you think, feel, want and need, whom to trust and whom to avoid, as well as what to do and when to do it. This is the wise part of you that already recognizes the insanity of our culture's obsession with thinness. It is also the place where you will discover a sense of meaning and purpose powerful enough to dispel the myth of fulfillment through thinness.

Practicing Cultural Criticism

Just as you need to practice being mindful to fully experience the power of the present moment and develop your ability to watch your inner experience, so too you have to practice cultural criticism to become adept at it. This takes time and effort. One of the easiest ways to begin is to scrutinize the popular media, which is ubiquitous. With the advent of the Internet and mass communications, you can hardly walk from one room of your house to the next (much less through a supermarket or across town) without catching a glimpse of an advertisement, magazine cover, or television program, each of which is usually rife with images and ideas that reflect The Religion of Thinness. With a little training it isn't so difficult to see that the messages broadcast by the media are often either outright lies or a subversion of deeper truths, many of which are sponsored by interested corporate entities whose continued wealth depends on your devotion.

Consider this advertisement from the *Self* magazine website:

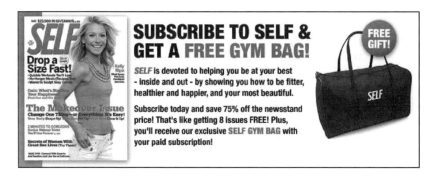

Advertisement from *Self* magazine website (March, 2008)

Let's take a few moments to analyze what it's *really* selling.

On the surface, the ad tells us that we will get a free gym bag with the purchase of a subscription to the magazine at a greatly discounted rate. It's quite a bargain. Too bad we have to buy so much other baggage along with it!

Before we even look at the text or the images, take a closer look at the free gym bag. Such a gift assumes that either we go to the gym or that we *should* go to the gym. Immediately, we are drawn into the world of health and fitness, which in our society are virtually synonymous with weight loss and thinness. After all, this is *Self*'s "Makeover

Issue," and the lead story is on dropping a dress size *fast*.

The magazine cover entices us with promises that are dubious at best. For example, *Self* will help us "Change One Thing—or Everything. It's Easy!" If you stop and think about it, this prospect is clearly ridiculous. Changing everything isn't easy—sometimes changing even one thing is downright difficult! Notice, too, how this enticement presumes that you want to change something (at least "one thing") about yourself, particularly some aspect of your appearance—your figure ("Shape Up!") or maybe your skin ("Clear it Up!")—as if renovating your body is the key to (re)defining your "self" and finding the satisfaction you seek.

A closer look at the advertisement's text confirms the link between happiness, health, beauty, and thinness. *Self* promises to help you "be at your best—inside and out—by showing you how to be fitter, healthier, and happier, and your most beautiful." Putting these terms together next to the model's slender body reinforces the notion that they are synonymous. Never mind that you don't need to be beautiful or thin by *Self* magazine's standards to be happy and healthy, or that being your best may consist of something entirely unrelated to your physical appearance

In fact, the very language of the ad reinforces the popular notion that how you look on the outside is an expression of your inner state. To be content on the inside you have to be "pretty" (read: thin) on the outside. That's why the magazine says it will show you how to achieve happiness, health, and beauty (e.g., through "Quickie Workouts" and "No Hunger Meals" that will help you "Sculpt Sexy Curves" or be "Gorgeous" in just "Two Minutes"). The emphasis here is really on appearance, despite the rhetoric about inner well-being.

If you think you have to go out of your way to find examples like these, you are sadly mistaken. When I first started studying media images of women about 20 years ago, I wondered if there would ever come a time when my cultural critiques would become unnecessary. Unfortunately, I have found the opposite to be true. Pop cultural pictures that glorify thinness are as pervasive as ever.

Throughout this book I present images from the mass media and help you deconstruct them as I just did to tease out the real messages they convey about food, weight, and your body. I also challenge the cultural paradigms and historical legacies underlying The Religion of Thinness. I hope this serves as a model to help you understand some of the ways the media and other sources of information exert their influence and lay the foundation for The Religion of Thinness to grow.

In fact, I suggest you make it a practice to analyze these kinds of images just as you make it a practice to sit and watch your breath. Make an effort to critically analyze the covers of magazines the next time you're waiting in line at the grocery store, the billboards you pass on the street, and the messages behind the pictures on the screen. Critique information you read in newspapers and other seemingly reliable sources. Reflect on every message you receive about your body and what it communicates about beauty, health, and success. Do the exercises that I offer in this book and you will take a large step toward being free from The Religion of Thinness.

The Mindful Cultural Critic: Linking One Practice to the Other

Cultural criticism helps us water the seeds of our inner wisdom by teaching us to think for ourselves. Yet it must engage more than our heads in order to give us a new sense of purpose. Intellectual understanding is not enough to shatter the myths that have shaped our beliefs and oriented our lives. To change our world view, our perspective must also enlist our emotions by engaging our hearts.

As we become more critically aware of our culture's storyline about the importance of our body size, we can also begin to be more mindful of the thoughts and feelings this narrative evokes within us. Our daily encounters with external images and messages about weight and eating can spark a host of internal reactions. A television ad for a weight-loss product stirs our desire to get our life back in control. A magazine cover asking, "Are You Too Fat?" throws us into a tailspin. A friend's passing comment, "You look so good! Have you lost weight?" elicits a sense of hope and achievement. Often, we're not even aware of the tides of these energies flowing within us, much less the extent to which our reactions are a result of cultural conditioning.

Becoming more aware of the relationship between the thoughts and feelings within us and the messages around us helps us understand the evolution of our body hatred. Knowing this doesn't make our reactions go away. But it can serve as an impetus for learning from them. Both "good" and "bad" feelings can become our teachers when we approach them with curiosity rather than judgment.

As you start to recognize the insanity of The Religion of Thinness, you don't need to judge yourself for having consumed the lies it fed you. We all consume them. It's almost impossible not to. But with practice you will begin to awaken from the stupor. As you do, use your new-found understanding of the illusion you have bought into as an opportunity to grow, not a means to further condemn yourself.

Remain mindful of your inner experiences. Observe them with compassion for yourself. Tread gently on this path to healing and deepening your spirit. With practice, you will tap more deeply into your real values, and this will make you less vulnerable to the untruths of The Religion of Thinness. Keep critiquing these untruths, and eventually you will become capable of trusting your inherent wisdom.

Practice – Not Perfection

The courage to begin the journey toward wholeness materializes when we take the first step. What prevents most of us from making this move is not that we don't want to, but that we don't know how to: love our bodies, eat when we're hungry, stop when we're satisfied, enjoy a meal without purging, see through the deceptions of The Religion of Thinness, and remain mindful of our inner reactions. Perhaps you are haunted by memories of trying but failing to do things differently. Perhaps you're paralyzed by doubt that your relationship with your body can ever change. Whatever your story, the only way to learn how to do something you've never done before is to practice.

Seeing recovery as an ongoing process, rather than something that needs to be accomplished once and for all, can make the first step seem less daunting. Healing is not about doing it "right." In fact, such an expectation sets you up for failure. The goal is not perfection. It's not even about "making peace" with your body because peace is a *process—an ongoing, evolving practice—not a final destination.*

There is no state of being "cured" and no magic bullet that will suddenly make things better. The pain, emptiness, and problems that cause us to seek salvation through a thinner body do not miraculously disappear just because we decide it's time to make changes. In the memoir of her struggle with anorexia and bulimia, Marya Hornbacher reflects, "I have not, nor will I ever, completely lose the longing for that something, that thing that I believe will fill an emptiness inside me." At the same time, she says it's possible to learn to live with this yearning for "that something" in ways that are not self-destructive. She concludes, "I have learned to understand the emptiness rather than fear it and fight it and continue the futile attempt to fill it."[20] We grow in our ability to accept, rather than avoid or fill, the caverns and cravings within us, as we learn to stay present to the very difficulties we think we can't handle.

Spiritual growth is not something that occurs in another place and time. It is a journey that begins here and now—right in the midst of our eating problems. When we begin to envision the meaning of our life beyond the goal of getting thinner, our torturous struggles with food and weight become opportunities for opening our hearts and renewing our spirits.

Such opportunities are present in every encounter we have with food. This is very good news! It means that every day, in fact, several times a day, we have a chance to do things differently. We can make decisions about what, whether, or how much to eat based on the true needs of our flesh, rather than what our culture tells us we should or shouldn't eat. We can learn to appreciate the beauty and strength of our one-of-a-kind physiques, rather than constantly berating ourselves for not looking like emaciated mannequins. This transformation will take effort. In a world that encourages and rewards thinness, practicing peace with our bodies is an ongoing challenge and spiritual adventure that unfolds little by little, step by step.

So make a choice. Take a step. Make a commitment within yourself to practice the techniques and concepts you are going to learn in this book. Your journey toward peace starts now, not tomorrow, not in some distant and imagined future when you are thin and life is perfect, but today. This instant. It is the only moment you will ever have. Choose to use it to fulfill your spirit, not deny your body.

My hope is that this book will help you do that. By learning how to become mindful and present to your inner experiences, you will create a new relationship with yourself and the world you inhabit. Learning how The Religion of Thinness functions will loosen its grip on you. Becoming critical of our culture and the messages it feeds you will help you move slowly away from its meanings, rituals, symbols, and iconography toward your own truth—one that is directed by what you want out of life and what you hope to contribute to the world, not by the illusory connection between slenderness and salvation. By changing the very paradigm by which you understand food and your body, you will move from The Religion of Thinness to practicing peace with your body, and experience the wholeness you were looking for in the first place.

2

FROM ILLUSION TO INSIGHT

Dispelling "The Myth of Thinness" and Creating a New Sense of Purpose

"May I help you?" The sugary voice of the salesclerk jolted Katie back to reality. She had been studying the same pair of jeans for the past ten minutes, alternating between holding them up against her body then putting them back on the pile.

"No, thanks. Just looking," Katie said politely. She moved on to the next pile. But she couldn't stop thinking about those jeans. They would be perfect for the upcoming party—if she could just lose five or ten pounds. She'd have to starve herself for several days, but maybe this was the incentive she needed to get back to her skinny-jean weight.

There it was again, that annoying, ever-present feeling that those extra pounds were preventing her from really living. Katie's obsession with losing weight bothered her almost as much as the weight itself. She found herself constantly thinking that if she were thinner, her life would be perfect. She recognized the absurdity of this belief, but that didn't make it less powerful. As she paid for the jeans, she felt a renewed sense of purpose. Maybe this time she really would do it.

What is it about the prospect of a slender body that is so alluring? Do you, like Katie, spend hours pondering what it would be like to fit into a special pair of jeans? Does the possibility of achieving this goal fill you with a sense of hope? Is there a part of you that believes you *can't* be happy, pretty, successful, or carefree *unless* you are thin?

The Myth of Thinness—the belief that thinness equals happiness, a primary tenet of The Religion of Thinness—disguises a much deeper longing for a meaningful and fulfilling life. It addresses our need for a sense of purpose, a calling or vocation that gives us direction and makes our days feel worthwhile. This longing is rooted in the fundamental mysteries of life: *Why are we here? Why do we suffer? How should we live? What happens when we die?* While no one can answer these "big" questions conclusively, we all need some kind of faith or worldview to orient our journeys through life's uncharted waters.

Religious and cultural narratives play a pivotal role in establishing the beliefs we have about our place in the cosmos. From the biblical story of Adam and Eve, Jews and Christians learn that humans find fulfillment in their relationship to a divine power who created all things. The Qur'an also has a version of this story that helps Muslims understand how they are free to exercise their own judgments but are also restrained by divinely imposed limits. Hindus believe that the distinction between Creator and creature is an illusion, because the sacred is manifest everywhere and in everything. Their tales of gods and goddesses illustrate the multiple ways in which seekers can come to know the divine. In Buddhism, the legend of Siddhartha's search for enlightenment points to the impermanence of life and suggests that letting go of attachments is the way to cultivate true peace and happiness.

Despite their differences, these symbolic stories—the myths—of established religions have a common function: they connect believers to a greater reality. Spiritual myths employ the power of metaphor to engage the imagination and stir emotions, speaking to us in ways that narratives based primarily on reason cannot. They become especially important during times of crisis or despair. They help us cope with life's various pressures—from traumatic experiences to everyday frustrations—by reminding us, at every level of our being, of the ultimate purpose of our lives. Like the myths of traditional religion, the basic storyline of The Myth of Thinness—*lose weight and you will be happy-pretty-successful-carefree*—provides a blueprint not just for how we should appear, but more importantly, how we should live.

This chapter explores this Myth of Thinness, offers a historical perspective, describes how it functions to define our purpose on a daily basis, and explains why it is so mesmerizing. Along the way I introduce techniques to become mindful and critical of this influential myth so you can break free from its power and move from illusion to insight.

The Myth of Thinness: How It Functions

Myths are not simply stories we *believe* in, they are stories we *dwell* in. We grow up surrounded by them, but we are often unaware of their power.

Those of you who were raised in a traditionally religious family, as I was, have a direct experience with this. If you grew up Christian, for example, you probably went to church on Christmas because that's when Christians celebrate the birth of Christ—God's entry into the world in human form. As a child, you probably didn't realize how the symbolic meanings of this story—the birth of hope in times of darkness, the presence of greatness in the form of a baby, the promise of deliverance from pain and affliction—shaped your orientation to life, enabling you to find something to hold onto in times of suffering throughout your life. You did not have to memorize these truths. You probably weren't even aware that you were learning them. They were part of the landscape that shaped your worldview through repeated exposure to the Christmas story. With time, the "truths" of such narratives become so deeply etched in your experience that they seem natural or universal rather than a product of a particular culture, tradition, and historical era.

This is how The Myth of Thinness gains adherents. Its omnipresence ensures that we absorb its meanings, even when we are not conscious of taking them in. Typically, the desire to lose weight begins slowly and subtly in response to self-consciousness about our bodies. Frequently there is some trigger event: a passing comment by a parent or friend, a painful name-calling incident on the playground, a physical change due to puberty. It can even grow out of the simple desire to fit in. Whatever the catalyst, many of us waste years feeling ashamed of and estranged from our physical selves as a result.

The shame we experience is created and reinforced by the endless messages surrounding us that we *should* be embarrassed about our "imperfect" bodies, and that the only way these feelings will be relieved is if we achieve the slender ideal. Advertisements for slimming products and programs are everywhere, promising a new life through a thinner you. Hope-inspiring testimonies about successful weight loss through dieting, exercise, drugs, hypnosis, liposuction, gastric by-pass, and every other conceivable method reinforce the illusion that fulfillment is just a few lost pounds away.

The pervasiveness of The Myth of Thinness gives it the aura of being a *fact*, rather than a socially-fabricated fiction. It goes without saying that thinner is better, and few dare to doubt this conventional "wisdom." As one average-sized college student said:

> There's no way you could convince me that my body is acceptable just as it is. Even people who are just a little overweight look unhealthy and unattractive to me. I'm always wishing I were thinner. Everyone knows that people who are skinny are happier, prettier, and better off in just about every way.

The monologues repeated in our heads are evidence of the extent to which this faith in slenderness has infiltrated our lives. "I would be happier if I lost weight" is a shared—though often unwitting—mantra that connects women who might otherwise have little in common. A few lucky individuals hear this voice only occasionally, but many hear it every day, some to the point of being unable to tune it out.

How did this happen? Women have not been plagued with obsessive thoughts about their weight since the birth of the human race. How then has The Myth of Thinness become so prevalent that it is rarely questioned? We need only look back at recent history for answers.

The Myth of Thinness in Historical Perspective

Had we lived over 100 years ago, things would have been significantly different. Until relatively recently, most people in the United States believed that thinness was unattractive and a sign of poverty or sickness. In the decades following the Civil War, for example, a voluptuous model of female beauty—epitomized by Lillian Russell—became widely popular.[1]

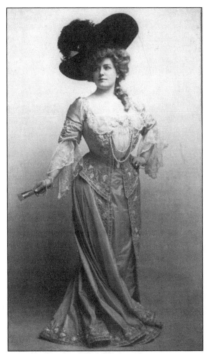

Lillian Russell, 1904 fashion photo

One writer of this period declared that, "plumpness is beautiful," and that, "great thinness, or as it is called *scragginess*… is no longer esteemed lovely." Another beauty adviser of the time recommended the full-figure ideal by citing the maxim that, "a sweet temper and a bony woman never dwell under the same roof."[2] For the wives of wealthy men, fat was considered a "silken layer."[3]

It was not until the early 1900s that a confluence of ideologies and institutions challenged the appeal of a well-cushioned female figure. At this time, the medical community decided that being plump indicated poor health. Needless to say, this view is still widely held today, despite evidence suggesting that being slightly to moderately overweight is not unhealthy, and that thinness is not necessarily a sign of vigor. In fact, a large 2008 study found that the death rate among "overweight" adults was lower than those of normal weight, although morbidly obese individuals had a higher rate.[4]

Insurance companies in the 1950s legitimized the medical bias against fat using data based on the lives of wealthy individuals (primarily men) to set standards for "ideal" weights.[5] Meanwhile, the fashion industry was shrinking the size of the "ideal" female figure. When Twiggy appeared on magazine covers in 1967, she stood 5' 7" and weighed a mere 91 pounds.[6] During the 1970s, the federal government issued a report called "Dietary Goals," which warned that Americans' overeating patterns "represent as critical a public-health concern as any before us."[7]

On the religious front, evangelical Christian authors wrote books like *Help Lord! The Devil Wants Me Fat*, which demonized obesity as a sign of depravity and insisted that God prefers us skinny.[8] I address the evangelical Christian dieting movement in more detail in Chapter 5, where I discuss The Morality of Thinness, and the dangers that are created when body size becomes an index of ethical behavior.

For now, it is important to understand that the *thinness = health & happiness* equation so many of us have grown up accepting as fact is not inherently true. We understand it as such because we have lived with this myth our whole lives. None of you reading this book grew up in the late 1800s when the idea that *plumpness = beautiful* was predominant. If you had, you likely wouldn't accept The Myth of Thinness as readily as you do and would probably consider large-bodied women to be beautiful. Instead, you grew up in a society where powerful institutions and ideologies such as the medical establishment, insurance companies, the fashion industry, and even certain religious movements have supported and promoted the idea that thinness equals health and happiness despite the fact that they do not automatically correlate.

In fact, because you were born and raised when you were, The Myth of Thinness has been woven into the fabric of your life. It's likely that you have accepted this myth (at least to some degree), even though rationally you know it can't be true. Like all modern women, you have been sold lies about your body by the diet entrepreneurs who launched a multi-billion dollar industry pedaling ways to eradicate "excess" flesh[9] and the commercially-sponsored mass media that spreads this message with missionary zeal.

Commercial Underpinnings of The Myth of Thinness: Diet Entrepreneurs and the Promises They Sell

As long as you remain unhappy with your body, someone stands to profit. Your discontent is an exploitable resource. And those who benefit are not primarily concerned with your well-being; they are far more interested in your money.[10] Weight-loss companies and marketers have helped shape and support The Myth of Thinness, because by doing so they can capitalize not only on your desire to be thinner but also on your deeper longing for a sense of purpose and self-worth.

As a way of refining our skills in cultural criticism, let's consider how top-selling weight loss programs are marketed. Let's start by looking at a banner that was used at NutriSystem's website in 2008. Although these images are routinely changed, this example is typical:

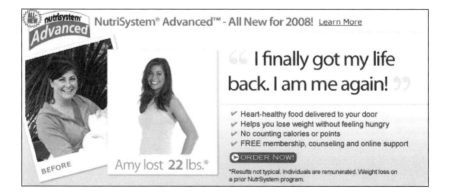

NutriSystem® home page banner

Could the promise of a reclaimed and joyful existence be more self-evident? NutriSystem doesn't just help you lose a few pounds; it will give your "*life* back." In fact, given the context and screen layout, the two concepts are interconnected. The photos are the first things we see. But we don't look at them in detail. Our eyes just pass over the image of Amy long enough to realize that she did indeed lose weight (22 pounds, the larger-font text under her "after" photo informs us). As we continue to peruse the ad, our eyes see the largest text in the banner, which exclaims, "I finally got my life back. I am me again!" Several ideas are now connected: Amy lost weight, as verified by her photos and the associated text; this is an "excellent" outcome not only because she appears more beautiful by our culture's dominant standards, but also because she got her life back by doing so; and NutriSystem could give *you* your life back too, if you "ORDER NOW!"

Notice that there is never a question about what it means to "get your life back." We all know. It means you would be happy, pretty, successful, and carefree. The fact that the meaning of these words is actually *not* self-evident is of little consequence because the ad appeals to us on an emotional level. It taps into our desire for happiness. It shows and tells us that losing weight leads to happiness, and that NutriSystem can help us lose weight/be happy. What more do we need to know?

Testimonials of this kind, where a seemingly-average person endorses the effectiveness of a particular weight-loss regimen, are commonplace in the diet industry. They usually speak to life changes that the program promises more than the weight it is designed to help you lose. They become acknowledgments of faith that marketers have found very successful in selling products like these.

What's interesting, however, is that many of these testimonials *don't* come from real people who have used the program. As it happens, this website is chock full of these types of before-and-after photos with the same, exact testimonial. Apparently many of the women who use this weight-loss program say the words, "I finally got my life back. I am me again!"

More astonishing is the barely-noticeable, minuscule text at the bottom of the banner. It refers to the asterisk next to Amy's weight loss figures and states, "Results not typical. Individuals are remunerated. Weight loss on a prior NutriSystem program." So, Amy is not an average person on the program after all. Her results are *unusual*. She was paid, possibly for the use of her pictures or to actually lose the weight. And the results she achieved were on a different NutriSystem program, not the "new" and "advanced" one this banner is selling. This kind of deceptive advertising (in which the professed message conflicts with the reality behind it) also conditions us to lie to ourselves, until we find ourselves embracing the myth that purchasing the product will change our lives.

An entire chapter could be devoted to deconstructing this advertisement, but the main points are as follows:

- The banner isn't ostensibly set up as an advertisement. It's simply the announcement that introduces the NutriSystem home page. This makes it seem as though it isn't selling you a product when, in fact, that is the *only* thing it is designed to do.

- Unlike the "before" picture, it is painfully clear that in her "after" picture, Amy is wearing an elegant dress, is tan, has make up on, her hair is down and has been colored and curled, and she is wearing tinted contact lenses that make her eyes appear bright blue.

- If you look closely you can see Amy is holding a *newborn baby* in her "before" photo. It's barely covered by the "after" shot. Is this Amy's baby? Did she lose those 22 pounds just after giving birth?

- Finally, the banner connotes that all of the wonderful benefits you could receive weren't available in 2007. The implication is that you are truly *fortunate* to have this amazing opportunity in front of you so you better hurry and "ORDER NOW."

I don't presume to tell you much that you don't already know about advertising. We are all aware that the photos are doctored and that the text can be misleading. In fact, you *know* this so well that you may even think advertisements like these have no effect on you. Most people feel this way. But if this were true, why does the weight loss industry spend billions of dollars a year promoting itself?[11] And why is this self-promotion so successful?

NutriSystem reported revenues of $777 million in 2007. Other conglomerates, like Jenny Craig® and WeightWatchers offer similar messages and have huge budgets. Jenny Craig, which is a subsidiary of Nestlé, has rotating banners with celebrities and "real people" proclaiming their weight loss, great health, and newfound happiness. They had $558 million revenue in 2007. The WeightWatchers website claims that, "Weight Watchers works because it's *not* a diet." But, it is all about weight loss. Consumers spent $4 billion on their products and services in 2007 alone.[12] A Google search for "diet products" produces nearly five million results. Weight loss is big business.

Women who subscribe to weight loss programs do so not because they lack intelligence, but because they sense that something is missing. Shedding pounds becomes a way to inject their lives with new energy and purpose, and diet marketers exploit this yearning.

In fact, the rhetoric in ads for diet programs often focuses more on transforming your life than reshaping your figure. The banner at the top of the Jenny Craig website reads: "Jenny Craig We Change Lives." It doesn't say "Jenny Craig We Help You Lose Weight." Rather, it promises something much more profound: a chance to be happy—to "get your life back" (NutriSystem) or to "Start Living" (Weight Watchers). Of course, the problem with these promises is that changing your life is not as simple as changing your body, and losing weight is not a reliable route to happiness.

More Commercial Underpinnings: Cashing in on Our Schizophrenic Relationship with Food

Corporations that sell the idea of a happier you through a thinner body are cashing in on the very dissatisfaction they help to generate and making *serious* amounts of money in the process. But what is downright maddening is that the same commercial interests that underwrite this mythical quest promote the kind of overeating and types of foods that have led so many people to *gain* weight in the first place. For example, Nestlé's riches come from selling candy. How convenient to also sell a weight loss program to remove the pounds those candy bars helped put on. Kraft Foods, producer of brands like Cheez Whiz, Chips Ahoy!, and Marshmallow Twirls also featured "South Beach Living" foods on its website in the spring of 2008. Visitors were invited to "Discover Kraft recipes and products that are recommended for the South Beach Diet."

The fast-paced growth of weight-loss industries in the second half of the 20th century paralleled the expanded manufacturing and marketing of highly-refined, sugary, salty, fatty, high-calorie foods. According to journalist Michael Pollan, these additives "push our evolutionary buttons"—our innate preference for certain tastes. But they do little to satisfy our nutritional needs, and this may be one reason we are prone to consume them in large quantities. In his book, *In Defense of Food*, Pollan quotes renowned biochemist Bruce Ames, who suggests that the insatiable hunger many people experience when eating highly processed foods, "may be a biological strategy for obtaining missing nutrients."[13] It makes sense that a body that is largely fed on sugar, salt, and fat is not getting sufficient nutrients and will be inclined to continue to feed in the hope of obtaining them.

No doubt the growing market for these foods has contributed to the highly-publicized, "obesity epidemic" in America today. In December 2003, *Newsweek* declared obesity to be "the biggest health crisis facing the country." Some studies indicate that two-thirds of American adults are overweight and that half of them are obese. The percentage of children who are seriously overweight (15 percent) has tripled since 1970.[14] The list of health problems that some studies link to excess weight—heart disease, diabetes, certain types of cancer, to name a few—is well publicized.

At least in part, our ever-expanding girth can be seen as a result of the schizophrenic messages we receive about weight and eating. While we are encouraged to abstain, restrict, or purge, we are also beckoned to indulge, dig in, and splurge. Ironically, these messages actually come from the same sources. Jenny Craig's website not only displays thin models, but places delicious looking cakes right next to them. Nutri-System has photos of chips, chili, and strudel on its site. Each of these companies sells these types of foods; in fact these are the "diet" foods on which the programs are based. Yet even a brief look at the list of ingredients on most of the products any of these three corporate giants sell reveals their nutritional or weight loss value to be questionable at best. They are filled with sugars and preservatives.

Consider NutriSystem's NutriFrosted Crunch Cereal, which contains five different sweeteners: high fructose corn syrup, evaporated cane juice, barley malt extract, sugar, and malt flavoring. High fructose corn syrup undergoes enzymatic processing to increase its fructose content and frequently is made from corn that has been genetically modified to withstand tremendous amounts of pesticides. The process for making this super-sugar, which was developed as an inexpensive domestic substitute for cane sugar, was perfected in the 1970s, after which it was incorporated in millions of processed foods and soft drinks worldwide.[15] In fact, there is a direct correlation between the rise of high fructose corn syrup in the U. S. food supply and the rise of obesity in this country. The average American consumed approximately 62.6 pounds of this highly processed substance in 2005.[16]

On the other hand, some cases of weight gain occur as a *result* of restrictive eating. The body adapts to caloric reduction by becoming more efficient at energy conservation, holding on to calories in its fat cells. This slowed metabolism makes it increasingly difficult to lose weight and frustratingly easy to put on the pounds. The body's ability to adjust to caloric deprivation explains why as many as 95 percent of people who initially lose weight on diets end up gaining back all the weight they lost—plus more—once normal eating is resumed.[17]

What's more, the same Americans who spend over $60 billion a year to lose weight are constantly bombarded with commercials enticing them to "supersize" what they eat.[18] A single meal at many popular restaurant chains often contains well over *half* the daily recommended calories for a healthy person. From the family-sized packaging of snacks and sodas to the mega-portions served at restaurants, Americans now eat 200 more calories per day than they did 10 years ago.[19]

There are *enormous* profits to be made from this cultural confusion about food and how we eat. It is no accident that the same companies that sell unhealthy, chemically-processed foods created to increase shelf life (and therefore increase their bottom line) sponsor The Myth of Thinness. Doing so gives them an extraordinary advantage in the market place: the opportunity to feed you cheaply-produced, oversized, fatty meals with one hand and diet programs with the other.

This schizophrenia is reflected in our attitudes toward exercise as well. As our waistlines continue to expand, we have become more sedentary than ever. Roughly 75 percent of adult Americans fail to meet even the minimal government advisements for daily exercise: 30 minutes of walking (or something equivalent). Thanks to an assortment of technological developments, most of us are living out of sync with our bodies' natural needs for movement. Our stationary habits affect not only our bodies (in terms of weight gain), but our spirits as well. Some experts believe that insufficient exercise is a major contributing factor in today's epidemic of mood and anxiety disorders, including depression. For some people, this leads to a vicious cycle of overeating to quell the depression, decreased activity because of weight gain, which leads to even more depression.[20]

Our sedentary ways increasingly start early. According to the Center for Disease Control, "walking and bicycling by children aged 5 to 15 dropped 40 percent between 1977 and 1995." Meanwhile, many schools are cutting physical education classes because they don't have the money to fund them.[21] The average child in the U.S. today spends five-and-a-half hours a day with some kind of electronic media (watching television, playing video games, using a computer, text messaging, etc.), most of which require very little physical activity. According to Steven Gortmaker of the Harvard School of Public Health, "the best single behavioral predictor of obesity in children and adults is the amount of television viewing."[22] Gortmaker's conclusion is that this correlation is not simply because watching TV burns very few calories, but rather the way advertisements affect viewers' decisions about how to spend their food dollars.

The Media's Missionary Role in Spreading
The Myth of Thinness

No matter what your size, the media affects how you feel about food and your body. And, because its audience is so vast, mass communications have the power to *normalize* the preference for the lean and svelte figure, making slenderness seem like the best shape for *every* body. The internet, magazines, books, television, popular movies, and all types of advertising contribute by unanimously promoting slim and sleek as the one and only desirable shape. These media outlets have a *cumulative* effect, making the desire to lose weight seem as natural as breathing. We live in the myth.

Let's consider the effects of television alone. About 99 percent of American families have television, and the average child grows up in a home with 3.5 television sets and watches an average of 25 hours per week. One in five spends as much as 44 hours per week in front of the set, and the majority of children ages 8 to 18 spend more time sitting in front of a television, computer, or game screen than any other activity in their lives except sleeping.[23]

A 1996 study found the amount of time an adolescent watches soaps, movies, and music videos is associated with his or her degree of body dissatisfaction and desire to be thin. Another study among undergraduates discovered that media consumption is positively associated with the pursuit of thinness among men and body dissatisfaction among women. And it comes as little surprise that teenage girls who watch commercials depicting unrealistically thin women report that they feel less confident, more angry, and more dissatisfied with their weight and appearance compared to those with less exposure to such images. It's also interesting to note that there are 16 minutes of advertising in the average hour of primetime television. In one study of Saturday morning toy commercials, analysts found that 50 percent of those directed at girls spoke about physical attractiveness.[24] This is the world we grow up in. Is there any wonder why we believe The Myth of Thinness? And of course this is only television. These false messages about weight and body image come from every conceivable media outlet, even the news.

Consider this cover of *U.S. News & World Report*. Although it appeared in the mid-1990s when The Myth of Thinness was rapidly gaining momentum, the concern it represents—whether you are "too fat"—is hardly a relic of the past. This particular example illustrates how the mainstream news media contributes to The Myth of Thinness through its presentation of "facts."

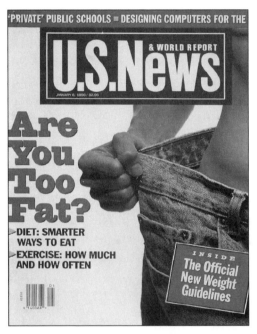

U.S. News & World Report: "Are You Too Fat?"

Would you ever question whether the "Official New Weight Guidelines" in *U.S. News & World Report* were an accurate assessment of what you "should" weigh? After all, such reports rely on scientific research. Still, this doesn't mean we should accept the "facts" they present without question—as if the scientific community were immune to our culture's enormous bias in favor of thinness. The image of a half-naked female body on the cover, which offers just enough of a glimpse of a woman's breast to catch our attention, should clue us in to the way "scientific" news stories can be influenced by cultural clichés. Even if such reporting were totally bias-free (an impossible prospect), should we automatically assume that its one-size-fits-all diagnoses, standards, and solutions apply to us? We might also question whether the information in such reports is truly newsworthy in a world afflicted by global problems like war, poverty, disease, and climate change.

In this context, it is particularly unfortunate that the West's preoccupation with thinness is also being exported to the global community. A widely-published study conducted in Fiji illustrates this influence. Prior to the introduction of television in 1995, this island nation had no reported cases of anorexia nervosa or bulimia and no outward signs of body-dissatisfaction. But just three years after American and British programs began broadcasting there, more than two-thirds of Fijian girls surveyed said they had attempted dieting to lose weight, and three-quarters of them said they felt "too fat." A study of Arab girls and women in London, England, and Cairo, Egypt, revealed a similar pattern: females who were exposed to the images and norms of Western culture were more likely to develop eating and body-image disturbances.[25]

There is also evidence that body dissatisfaction is increasing among women in India. Shikha Sharma is a medical doctor-turned-dietitian who runs a commercial weight-loss program in a South Delhi colony. Her clients range from young girls to women in their 70s—all of them seeking to reduce the size of their bodies. An increasing number are already thin, and occasionally anorexic women come to her looking for help with losing even more weight. One 2001 study revealed early signs of anorexia nervosa and bulimia in many of the 450 college students surveyed in Mumbai. Another Mumbai-based study of an elite college in that city found 40 percent of the female respondents to be malnourished by World Health Organization standards. The fact that Indian girls from well-off families are showing signs of malnutrition points to excessive dieting that is media-induced, according to Dr. Sadikote, author of the second study.[26]

The global influence of America's mandate for female slenderness is evident in contemporary women's magazines around the world, as well. The cover of an Indian edition of *Elle* displays a provocatively dressed, bone-thin woman alongside the titles "Are You a Fat-Skinny?"

and "Under the Skin of Cellulite." A seemingly more traditional Indian women's magazine, *Femina*, shows the frail face of a young woman on the cover, next to the heading: "Jeans Against Cellulite: Boost Your Hip Appeal." Articles like "Fast-Track to a Flat Stomach," "From Flab to Fab!" and "2 New Ways to Shed Kilos" line the front of a South African issue of *Shape*, which also features a slender, white, bikini-posing model. Through their shared focus on thinness, many of the popular women's magazines that circulate in Third World countries are virtually indistinguishable from their counterparts in the U.S.[27]

Eating disorders, the extreme outcome of The Religion of Thinness, occur globally; and, as in the United States and Western Europe, prevalence rates increased since the 1970s. In Japan, the number of patients in treatment for anorexia nervosa doubled between 1976 and 1981 and more than quadrupled by 1992. At that same time, slightly more than 1 percent of students surveyed in mainland China suffered from bulimia and 78 percent of the females feared weight gain. By the early 90s, eating disorders were reported in 37 countries, including such diverse places as Chile, Egypt, Iran, Nigeria, South Africa, and Turkey. They are also found in Central and Eastern Europe.[28]

What is perhaps most disturbing about cases like these is that most of these cultures, including our own, traditionally favored full-bodied, voluptuous women. The missionary impulse of the media and The Myth of Thinness that it promotes is reshaping these cultures' norms to match the West's expectations. This impulse is akin to that of religious groups that seek to convert non-believers and bring them into the fold. The media's proselytizing influence may not be as blatant as the church's historic power to indoctrinate, but the methods it uses to convert people to The Religion of Thinness are strikingly similar. Both:

- Provide role models by which people are encouraged to shape their lives

- Create a sense of order and purpose

- Shape people's sense of self and reality by teaching them what to value, how to behave, and of course, how to look

- Presume the convert needs something he or she doesn't already have

Given the preponderance of messages we receive from childhood onward teaching us that we can't be happy if we aren't thin, the power of the institutions that sponsor and support this belief, and the way they pass it off as "fact," it's little wonder that so many of us have accepted The Myth of Thinness as truth. In fact, many of us have subscribed to this myth so faithfully that thinness has *become* our primary goal in life.

Our Ultimate Purpose: Awakening from The Myth of Thinness

You probably do not *consciously* define your life's purpose according to The Myth of Thinness. If asked what you most value, the list would most likely include things like God, your health, love and compassion, inner peace, and your family. Few of us would respond that the size and shape of our figure is what truly matters. But in our everyday thoughts and actions, the possibility of being thinner may in fact *function* as our most cherished value and most precious ambition.

However limiting it seems, the goal of being thin can become our ultimate purpose when we lose sight of how our lives matter in the greater scheme of things. When it seems as though we are drifting aimlessly, this goal provides an anchor. If we feel powerless or insignificant, every encounter with food becomes an opportunity to achieve something. The sense of purpose you derive from renovating your body may help you avoid situations that make you feel anxious—work-related stress, a difficult marriage, a controlling parent or a troubled child. If you feel depressed, unsatisfied, or lonely, you may use your pursuit of a slender body as a salve for your pain.

Different women adopt The Myth of Thinness for different reasons. Your reasons are your own. But whatever the case, I would guess that compared to the larger issues in your life (those that lack easy answers), the "problem" of your body has a solution that seems alluringly un-complicated and attainable. This is one reason so many of us become converts. It appeals to our desire to accomplish something; and, not only does the outcome seem possible (because we are constantly told we can achieve it), but we also believe that by achieving it, all our other problems will go away.

Believing "I'm too fat" allows a woman to redirect her angst into a manageably small but all-consuming challenge: to contain her appetites and reshape her body. Reflecting back on her struggle with anorexia and bulimia, Abra Fortune Chernik wrote:

> Controlling my body yielded an illusion of control over my life.... I had reduced my world to a plate of steamed carrots, and over this tiny kingdom I proudly crowned myself queen."[29]

Despite the sense of power it temporarily yields, despite its alluring simplicity and promise to help you accomplish something, deep down, you know that The Religion of Thinness is not fulfilling your most important needs. In fact, you would probably choose to stop thinking about weight and calories—if only you could. But the sense of purpose that striving to be thin gives us is incredibly hard to give up no matter how empty it ultimately is. One woman who struggled for years with anorexia nervosa recalled the difficulty she had relinquishing her obses-sion with thinness:

> It's hard to let go of the one thing that makes you feel like you've really accomplished something. I was tired of thinking about my body all the time, but I couldn't stop because losing weight was something I knew I could always work towards. Sure, I had other dreams, like going to law school and getting married. But they were not as simple and immediate as the goal of being skin-ny. I used this goal to motivate myself every day, throughout the day, especially when my life felt overwhelming or pointless.

This human need is so strong that we will create a false purpose, even one that is self-destructive. When we lose touch with what really gives our life meaning, or when we don't have the resources or emotional strength to pursue our true calling, we latch onto superficial cultural goals—like having a "good" body—to feel as though we've achieved something important. Letting go of this hollow goal is all but impossible if we do not get in touch with what will truly fulfill us.

What is Our Deeper Purpose?

What is truly fulfilling? What is your "calling" in life?

Spiritual teacher Eckhart Tolle offers a helpful way of exploring this question. He distinguishes between an "outer purpose," which is what you do with your life on a daily basis (i.e., your job, relationships, interests, etc.), and an "inner purpose," which is to awaken spiritually. On the outer level, your particular talents, values, and experiences make you unique. On an inner level, however, everyone shares a common purpose: to grow spiritually by being more present to and aware of your own life in relation to something universal. That is done by practicing methods to expand your heart, mind, and soul in ways that bring peace to your life and the lives of others.[30]

Letting go of an outer purpose that is as artificial as the goal of thinness and replacing it with inner peace should be an appealing notion. If the ideas in this book resonate within you, chances are that you are ready to explore your inner purpose more intentionally. It might be helpful to remind yourself that the fulfillment you get from losing weight is always short lived, and that The Myth of Thinness is a dysfunctional illusion that has held you back from reaching your potential for far too long.

Awakening to your true calling in life doesn't happen sometime in the future. It's not a matter of being spiritually evolved enough to start the journey. We can't wait. Even with our fears, we must start this process today, because *right now* is the only moment we will ever have. It is in this moment that we can find the inner peace and sense of connection to something greater that we seek.

Mindfulness: A Pathway into the Now

Practicing mindfulness is a pathway into the now, one that allows us to bring our sadness, stress, anxieties, and imperfections with us as we strive to wake up to our life's larger purpose and experience the happiness we seek.

Many of us have been seduced by The Myth of Thinness because we weren't paying enough attention to how its storyline appealed to our desire to accomplish something with our lives. Becoming mindful of what's going on in our bodies, feelings, thoughts, behaviors, and the world around us enables us to avoid doing further harm.

Mindfulness also makes us conscious of the fundamentally interconnected nature of reality. "This is like this, because that is like that," to borrow a phrase from Thich Nhat Hanh.[31] This insight helps us understand how our obsessions developed out of our spiritual need for a sense of purpose and in response to our culture's die-hard devotion to thinness. Practicing mindfulness moves us from illusion to insight by opening our eyes to the pivotal role that cultural conditioning plays in the development of eating problems. It helps move us out of the semi-hypnotic state in which we so often move through the world, and enables us to see clearly the vast social influences that convince us our bodies need perpetual improvement. Becoming conscious of the beliefs we have internalized loosens their grip on us.

To help you begin to awaken from The Myth of Thinness, I would like you to try a mindfulness exercise called, "Watching the Watcher." It is designed to help you become more aware of your responses to the messages at the heart of this myth, without attaching to them.

In this exercise, I will ask you to *deliberately* expose yourself to an example from the media that promotes The Myth of Thinness, and then sit and become mindful of the thoughts, feelings, and bodily sensations that come up as a result. Please note that the purpose of this is *not* to create another opportunity to beat yourself up for not having the "perfect body," but to decrease the media's power to influence you by becoming more conscious of your internal reactions to it.

To do this, you need to step back and take the perspective of the "observer self" (that part of you that is able to watch your internal experience without judgment) and simply see what comes up when you encounter images or stories that support The Myth of Thinness. Follow these steps:

Step One: Pick an image or media story

First, locate an example from the media that promotes The Myth of Thinness. Doing this shouldn't be too difficult. Pick up a magazine or newspaper, turn on the television, or log on to the Internet and you will find a multitude of appropriate possibilities. Briefly study it.

Step Two: Sit with your thoughts and feelings

After looking at and/or reading your chosen image or text, find a comfortable and quiet place to sit and observe the inevitable mental response that will surface. Take at least five minutes. Keep your back straight, breathe from your belly, count your breaths (if you wish), and be still. Simply watch your internal reactions (mental, emotional, physical). Don't worry about the content of your reactions and whether they are "right" or "wrong." Just observing is enough. This piece is key: allow thoughts and emotions about your body to come and go naturally, without judgment or attachment. You are not trying to stop yourself from thinking or feeling, nor are you trying to explore your thoughts and feelings more deeply. You are simply watching them in order to "see" them more clearly.

Step Three: Float your thoughts down the river

To help you let go of your thoughts as they come up, imagine a long flowing river of crystal clear water. Trees line the borders of this magnificent work of creation. You can't stop the flow of the river. You can't push it to go faster. It simply flows on eternally. Every time a thought, feeling, or bodily sensation comes up, imagine writing it down on a leaf or piece of paper, release it into the river, and let it drift away with the current. Each time you do this, remember to come back to the present: the here and now.

This part of the exercise will help you realize that the thoughts you are having in response to your chosen text or image—"Look at her flat stomach compared to mine," "This diet looks easy enough," "I've got to get back in control," "If my legs were *that* thin"—are just that: *thoughts*. While they seem to be telling you the "real" story, in actuality they are more like the scenes from a movie you have been watching your whole life. The storyline of this drama is seductively simple: lose weight and you will be happy. However, the practice of mindfully watching your reactions to this drama helps you to see that socialized responses to cultural myths are no more "real" than the imaginary river you are using to float them away. This understanding is a crucial part of the movement from illusion to insight.

Step Four: Critique the messages

Finally, spend some time analyzing and deconstructing your image or story. Note that we are now shifting from mindfulness practice (simply watching what thoughts and feelings come up) to cultural critique (where we consciously engage with the media we have consumed). Be critical! You might ask yourself questions like these:

- What aspects of the image or story reflect The Myth of Thinness? For example: a smiling, ultra-thin model or a report on the "proven" health benefits of the latest diet.

- How does it draw the viewer in? Does it use flashy colors, bold printing, stereotypical images, or a particular arrangement of text and photos to lure your attention?

- What *obvious* ways does the text or image link happiness and thinness? Does it make blatant enticements that promise you more joy and vitality once you lose weight?

- What *less obvious* ways does the text or image create these associations? If you're looking at an ad featuring a slender woman, for example, is there a handsome man looking covetously at her? Is she sitting in a luxurious room, wearing expensive-looking clothes, or relaxing in a bikini on a beach?

- Who is really benefiting or profiting from the image or story you've been looking at? The question is fairly easy to answer if you've been looking at a commercial for a weight-loss product or program, but it can also be applied to other genre of media as well.

Whenever you encounter The Myth of Thinness, you can practice "Watching the Watcher" by pausing long enough to observe your internal reactions and send them down the river. The first few times you try this exercise might feel awkward. Waking up, becoming mindful, and getting present all take conscious effort, but every worthwhile journey begins with one step.

* * *

Many people come to a spiritual path in life because they are unhappy. What they often discover is that this very unhappiness offers enormous possibilities for personal growth. Our suffering has the potential to transform us. It can open our minds, expand our hearts, and free our spirits—*if we have the courage to be present to it*. Pain itself will not change us. But becoming conscious of our pain, sitting with it, getting to know it, and eventually letting go can help to wake us up spiritually. As the Franciscan priest Richard Rohr points out, "Spirituality is what we *do* with our pain."[32] It is a transformative process that requires our patience, persistence, and bravery.

When your efforts to dispel The Myth of Thinness seem to hit a roadblock, it's easy to feel discouraged. Just as we have adopted an idea of how our bodies are *supposed* to look, we may harbor ideas about how our healing is *supposed* to go. We want it to be clear, quick, and easy, and it seldom is. You may feel exhausted by your attempts to overcome the social conditioning you have lived with for decades. You may get depressed when change doesn't happen right away. You may even be tempted to add another layer of self-loathing to your already tormented self-image, especially if you interpret setbacks as failures to live up to some spiritual ideal.

When you find yourself disheartened in your efforts to heal, it's more important than ever to be patient with yourself and remember that the difficulties you encounter contain opportunities for growth. Every time you find yourself obsessing is a chance to practice being mindful. Pema Chödrön offers these words to those who are struggling on the path to greater self-awareness.

> We don't have to criticize ourselves when we fail, even for a moment, because we're just completely typical human beings; the only thing that's unique about us is that we're brave enough to go into these things more deeply and explore beneath our surface reaction of trying to get solid ground under our feet.[33]

Every time you fall back into old body-bashing habits, you have the chance to put mindfulness into practice. Please remember to:

1. Recognize how your desire to be thinner points to your need for a larger sense of purpose in life.

2. Spend time reflecting on how you envision this larger purpose. Investigate your most sacred values and what you want to accomplish during your lifetime.

3. Critically examine how our culture teaches you that losing weight will make you happier, and question the ways it encourages you to pursue thinness.

4. Reflect on the extent to which you've internalized the goal of thinness and the myth that losing weight will make you happy.

5. Practice mindfulness by noticing your internal responses to the media.

6. Let go of these internal responses by "floating your thoughts down the river."

7. Be patient when you find yourself drawn into The Myth of Thinness, and—without judging yourself—simply return to the present moment.

8. Have the courage to see your obsessive thoughts and behaviors not as signs of failure but as opportunities for spiritual growth.

Further Opportunities for Growth:
Dealing with Anger

Every difficulty you encounter on your journey of healing is yet another chance to be kind to your body and realign yourself with your life's larger purpose. Every time you catch yourself slipping back into your preoccupation with weight or eating, you are already waking up. In fact, the very moment you realize that you've been obsessing again is a moment of enlightenment. This is how you begin to deprogram yourself from The Myth of Thinness and move from illusion to insight.

As you do, any number of uncomfortable feelings may emerge, and one of the most challenging of these is anger. You may be angry either with yourself for having bought into the myth that thinness will make you happy or with society for promoting this lie. Anger is a difficult feeling for many women, because as girls we were taught to be accommodating and sweet—whatever the circumstances. Such gender training not only makes it hard to feel angry as adults, it also makes it difficult to criticize anything but ourselves. You don't risk losing someone's approval when you ridicule your expanding waistline, but if you critique a movie for depicting women as beautiful but brainless creatures, others might find you annoying or accuse you of spoiling the fun. We receive plenty of cues from the media, our families, and even our friends that nobody likes an angry woman.

Regardless of how you're perceived, anger may actually be a healthy response to the myths and belief that encourage your obsession with weight. Companies that promote and exploit our feelings of shame should make us mad. Images that convey a singularly narrow vision of health and beauty deserve our critique. We should take offense at advertisements that suggest our appetites cannot be trusted. We are being used by industries that capitalize on our spiritual yearnings by promoting weight loss as our ultimate purpose, and this ought to irritate us.

However, our anger need not turn into resentment. Rather, if we remain mindful and pay attention to this feeling, without being consumed by it, we can see how it is rooted in the pain The Myth of Thinness has caused us: the pain of feeling inadequate and unworthy because our bodies were less than "perfect"; the pain of seeing relationships destroyed because of our obsession; the pain of constantly postponing our lives until we lost weight; the pain of being trapped in our own little world of diet plans, scales, and calories. By using mindfulness and connecting this practice with cultural criticism, we can transform and harness the energy of our anger and use it as a motivating force that propels us to challenge and change our narrow-minded culture.

Changing Society by Making New Choices

The inner work we do prepares us to move towards transforming and awakening our society. Hence our outer purpose shifts from the pursuit of the perfect body to the pursuit of an awakened world, and becomes aligned with our inner purpose. This is the beginning of true happiness.

There's no question that this work is not nearly as simple-minded as going on a diet, but its satisfaction is far deeper and more enduring. Fortunately, change begins with the seemingly small, individual choices we make on a daily basis, like:

- Protesting the media's glamorization of thinness by sharing our viewpoint with our family and friends

- Refusing to purchase magazines that leave us feeling depressed and unworthy

- Turning off our television sets more often and refusing to support the messages they send us about food and our bodies

- Not going to commercial gyms that equate fitness with slenderness

- No longer buying weight-loss products that prey on our insecurities, or foods that encourage overeating

- Boycotting companies that use anorexic models or adult mannequins with waists the size of seven-year-old girls

- Writing letters of protest and making phone calls to companies that promote The Myth of Thinness

Try following the lead of a recovering bulimic woman who explained:

> The other day I received a mail-order catalog for women's clothing and on the cover were two models who looked like they hadn't eaten in weeks. I didn't even look inside the catalog but went straight for the phone, dialed the 800 number on the cover, and proceeded to tell the woman on the other end how much images of models like these have been hurtful to me. I made sure to be polite and not accuse her personally, and she not only listened dutifully to my complaint, but actually agreed with me and promised she would tell her supervisor about my call. It was such a simple act—it took less than five minutes—but I felt so empowered by the time I hung up.

In the course of our transformation, it's vital that we share our insights with others and find resources that support our shifting paradigm. Teaching mindfulness and cultural criticism to a younger generation of women—especially adolescent girls who are the most vulnerable prospective converts to The Religion of Thinness—is an important, positive step. There are an increasing number of resources to help us be mentors. Mind on the Media (www.mindonthemedia.org) is a national organization dedicated to "inspiring independent thinking and fostering critical analysis of media messages."[34] Through their "Turn Beauty Inside Out" program, they empower boys and girls to begin grassroots discussions, and sponsor events in their communities to increase awareness of the media's influence on girls' development. Similarly, the Girls, Women + Media Project (*www.mediaandwomen.org*) sponsors "I-CAN" (Involved Consumers Action Network), which offers information about consumer issues related to women and girls, and suggestions on how to take action. *New Moon* magazine (*www.newmoon.org*) is a publication for girls ages 8 to 14 that supports the development of their creative voices and critical skills. It is free of advertisements and is edited by the girls themselves.

Transform your self and you affect the world. This is what happens as you wake up from The Myth of Thinness. This is your purpose. It is an ongoing process, less about getting to the finish line than becoming who you are every day. It's a practice, not a product. And if you are persistent, change will happen, little by little, experience by experience. Each day you practice mindfulness, critique cultural messages, and challenge the powers that support The Religion of Thinness is a day you engage in the process of awakening. Each day spent this way is an investment in a happiness much more profound than weight loss can give you.

3

FROM IDOLATRY TO INSPIRATION

Seeing Through "The Icons of Thinness" and Finding New Sources for Self-Definition

Amy had already finished half of her popcorn by the time the previews were over. Grateful for the anonymity of the dark theater, she relaxed into her seat as the movie started. But the relaxation was short lived, because now Amy sat there, hand-to-mouth, studying the actress and her striking body. She noted the angular lines of her jaw and cheekbones, her elegant neck and endless legs. How could anyone be so thin?

Amy resolved again to start dieting tomorrow. She fantasized about how happy her life would be once she could control her need to eat. No longer enslaved by her bottomless hunger, she would be a stellar employee at work; she would feel sexy once again; she would have energy to burn; she would be the envy of others when walking down the street. Most importantly, she would finally be thin, and that would make her free—free from all her problems, including the endless battle with her weight, to eat what she liked when she liked, free from this body that had betrayed her by being so lumpy—to be just like that actress on the screen.

Like Amy, many of us have found ourselves staring enviously at the bodies of starlets and models, coveting the willpower we assume they possess, fantasizing about the admiration we know they enjoy, and desperately wishing we could look like them. Our misguided veneration is key to The Religion of Thinness. We bow down before the altar of thinness and its "graven images." In essence, we *worship* them. They are our modern-day icons, and though many of us are not consciously aware of their power, The Religion of Thinness relies on them to maintain its pull on us.

Every religion has sacred symbols and images that represent its highest values. So, too, the icons of The Religion of Thinness portray its most important ideal: thinness. The flawless body is our Mecca, our Canaan, our promised land. *The Icons of Thinness* become our guiding lights, illuminating our path to the physical perfection we seek.

However, beneath our idolization of slender women lies a deeper need for images that inspire our quest to define ourselves and realize our true potential. Each of us needs to have our spirits enlivened. We need visual guides to remind us of what we deem sacred, capturing our imaginations and calling forth the creative power within us. For when the visible images by which we frame our lives connect us to our deepest values, they keep our minds sharp and our hearts open, clarifying our ultimate purpose. When we orient our lives using our true aspirations, superficial fantasies cannot so easily seduce us.

As much as we may idolize them, The Icons of Thinness do not inspire and orient us this way. Rather than call forth our inner potential, they leave us feeling depressed, ashamed, and preoccupied with fixing our physical "flaws." They twist our perceptions of who we are and who we most *want* to be, leading us away from our true path. They are more like demons than demigods, because they draw us ever deeper into the web of deception fostered by The Religion of Thinness.

This chapter explains why images are important to us and examines how popular cultural iconography distorts and exploits our self-perception. It questions the narrow ideal that defines what it means to be a valued woman, and exposes society's demeaning messages, the elitism they presume, and the idolatry they promote. These discussions will prepare us to take another crucial step on our journey of recovery: finding and creating icons that nourish our spirits, in whose reflection we discover the motivation and courage we need to be whole and live peacefully inside our own skin.

Our Need for Inspiration: The Role of Icons

For most of human history, one function of religions was to provide images to inspire and orient humans in their search for wholeness. These sacred symbols, or icons, direct the attention of believers beyond daily existence toward that which promises to enlighten or fulfill. Religious iconography differs from ordinary images because its visual depictions are meant to point to a higher truth, and we are culturally conditioned to understand and respond to them in certain ways.

For example, the voluptuous and life-affirming statuettes of goddesses in ancient Neolithic cultures, such as the Venus of Willendorf, symbolized the fertile and mysterious powers of nature, reminding devotees to respect the earth and its cycles. It is likely that most modern viewers would not interpret the image this way—look at it and note your own reaction.

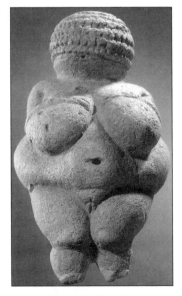

Venus of Willendorf

Similarly, Christians look to images of Jesus as loving teacher, sacrificial lamb, and a symbol of everlasting life, all of which foster courage and hope in the face of life's most difficult situations. The lotus flower, rising above its muddy roots to blossom in the sunlight, informs Buddhists to detach from the shifting waters of experience and be present to the beauty and perfection of life as it is. Each of these icons represents a particular set of truths that devotees are trained to understand in a particular way.

However, these icons do not have to be interpreted in this way. A picture of a lotus may just be seen as a beautiful flower to you, and a non-Christian does not think of Jesus as the Son of God. We interpret such images according to our own needs and background.

Despite the rather lofty ideals to which sacred symbols point, their function is simple and practical: they serve as visual reminders of an ultimate purpose, inspiring believers to strive to realize their highest calling. In Eastern Orthodox Churches, for example, icons of Jesus, Mary, and the saints painted in rich, glowing colors make present the reality of God in all of us and encourage believers to cultivate the qualities embodied in the persons depicted, such as compassion, humility, and wisdom. As vehicles for self-realization, such icons motivate their users by revealing the gap between who they are and who they could be. If religious myths establish the world views through which believers understand their life's purpose as described in the previous chapter, the sacred images these myths generate provide the inspiration needed to live out that purpose.

Just as The Religion of Thinness has its own mythology, so too it has its own set of sacred images to inspire and instruct our crusade for a different body. These images seduce us by creating an ideal that spurs us to reach beyond the limits of our ordinary life. The well-defined contours of their slim bodies stir our creative energies by inferring that the flawless body is attainable for each of us with a little stamina and the correct technique. Such physiques captivate our imaginations, because we have learned to see them as incarnating the extra-ordinary beauty, truth, and goodness we long to cultivate in ourselves. And despite the fact that these images are ultimately false gods (or goddesses) that lead us away from our true purpose, they still have incredible power to shape our perceptions—both of ourselves and of the women around us.

The Power of The Icons of Thinness and the Problems It Creates

Although we are constantly inundated with images in today's world, many of us don't realize their formative power. Unlike medieval Christians, for example, who consciously sought inspiration and personal transformation from representations of saints, many of us today encounter thousands of visual images without being aware of the lessons they instill.[1] Because we normally look at models and movie stars for entertainment, we tend to disregard the fact that their appearance communicates something— that we *should* be thin, and that we can't be happy, beautiful, or loved until we are.

It is precisely this *lack of attention* to how we are influenced by the media that makes us all the more susceptible to its subtle authority. And if you don't believe you are influenced by The Icons of Thinness, consider the following.

Studies have shown the negative effects of model-thin icons on female body image. A 1999 survey sponsored by Harvard Medical School found that 69 percent of girls between grades 5 and 12 admitted that fashion magazines influenced their perception of the ideal body. Among the 548 girls surveyed for this study, 66 percent said they wanted to lose weight, although only 29 percent of that group would be considered overweight by medical standards.[2] According to studies conducted at Stanford University and the University of Massachusetts, about 70 percent of the female co-eds who were interviewed said they felt worse about their appearances after looking at women's magazines. Additional research suggests that virtually all women tend to rate themselves as less attractive after viewing pictures of models.[3] Not surprisingly, men who have been studied react in similar ways.

Disturbing comments echo the findings above. "I *hate* how the magazines always have the prettiest, skinniest girls in them!" a 13-year-old girl exclaimed. "They make you feel so fat and ugly." This is a sentiment many of us share, but ironically we still don't make the connections—not because we are stupid—but because we are trained *not* to see through the veil of these images and deconstruct their inner meaning. Young women are particularly unaware. A 15-year-old bulimic girl who confessed she reads *Seventeen* magazine "like a Bible" said she'd never thought about the way the glossy photographs contributed to her own body-hatred. Instead of interpreting the models as unhealthy and unrealistic, she accepted them as "normal" and berated herself for her larger size.

Iconography's true function should be to inspire believers, to help them reflect on, cultivate, and live with high values. We look at spiritual images to motivate us to strive for peace, enlightenment, and a feeling of wholeness. But The Icons of Thinness almost always have the *opposite* effect. They have the uncanny ability to make us feel as though there's something wrong with our bodies, and by extension, ourselves. Rather than criticizing the messages these glossy pictures deliver, we learn only to criticize ourselves.

Why?

Omnipresence Equals Omnipotence

At least in part, our failure to scrutinize the media's glamorous portrayals of bone-thin women and the messages embedded in them is a consequence of their omnipresence. Depictions of doll-like, long-legged women are everywhere, visually reminding us of the absolute importance of being thin. Thanks to the technological advances of the past few decades, such reminders are more obvious than ever. Computers and a range of other electronic media—video games, iPods, and even some cell phones—widen our exposure. Those of us who read the daily news online can hardly avoid the endless pictures that idealize thinness. Indeed, there has never been a time on earth when media images were more abundant.

The ubiquity of the media has two important effects that further empower The Religion of Thinness and, by doing so, complicate our ability to be free from its influence: it reinforces the stereotypical association between women and the body, and it encourages us to understand, experience, and relate to our bodies through the lens of the photographs we consume.

Reinforcing the Historical Association Between Women and the Body

Hidden in the media's idealization of thinness is the time-worn assumption that, as women, we primarily define ourselves through our bodies (not our minds or hearts) and that how we look is both our most precious resource and our most probable downfall. In Western societies, cultural norms and religious traditions have routinely defined women by their bodies, whereas men have been characterized as rational and spiritual. In Christianity in particular, women have been depicted as more carnal than men because of insufficient reason, greater susceptibility to bodily cravings, and their role in leading men into temptation.

Ambrose, a 4[th]century church Father, illustrated this view in his interpretation of the story of the Fall of Humanity: the serpent represents the body's sinful pleasures; Eve represents our physical cravings; Adam represents both mind and spirit. In the eyes of Saint Augustine (354-430 CE), one of the most influential thinkers in the history of Christianity, Eve's fateful act demonstrates woman's "small intelligence," as well as her corresponding tendency to live "more in accordance with the promptings of the inferior flesh."[4] Erasmus of Rotterdam, a church reformer and Christian humanist during the Renaissance, echoed these associations over 1,000 years later:

> That slimy snake, the first betrayer of our peace and the father of restlessness, never ceases to watch and lie in wait beneath the heel of a woman, whom he once poisoned. By 'woman' we mean, of course, the carnal or sensual part of man. For this is our Eve, through whom the crafty serpent entices and lures our minds to deadly pleasures.[5]

Contemporary images that glamorize thinness recycle and perpetuate this historical standard by making women's physical form the focal point of their identity. From an early age, popular cultural images teach women that *how they look* exemplifies *who they are* and how they will be judged. This idea that the value of a woman is primarily contingent on her physical appearance, not on any of her other talents or attributes, is endlessly reinforced in our society. In point of fact, women's bodies are not only the basis for developing their sense of identity and worth; they are also a means for obtaining and exercising power. Author and activist Danzy Senna reflects on the different kinds of power women acquire in relation to their appearance, recalling that as a young girl she deliberated over which kind she wanted to cultivate in herself:

> There was the kind of power women got from being sexually desired, and the kind women got from being sexually invisible— that is, the power in attracting men and the power in being free of men. I also noticed that women fought one another for the first kind and came together for the second. Even as a child, I knew people craved power. I just wasn't sure which kind I wanted.[6]

So many women face this same challenge growing up. As a young woman, did you want to be sexually enticing or sexually invisible? Most of us can relate to one of these polarized options. The irony, of course, is that both kinds of power are associated exclusively with the body, as though other options for defining yourself (such as creative, intellectual, or spiritual pursuits) don't exist.

The quest for thinness also serves as a means for exercising certain "manly" virtues—especially autonomy and self-control—and by doing so enables women to transcend the confines of their fleshy existence. Such masculine qualities are displayed through the boyish figures of anorexic-looking models and actresses. Recalling the years she spent in a vicious cycle of starving and bingeing, one young woman describes the mentality and associations that fed her behavior.

> I never really liked having a female body. I mean, if you just look at most women's bodies, they look so out-of-control. You know, the big thighs, flabby arms, and wrinkles? I've always admired the kind of self-confidence and freedom that men seem to enjoy, and this is what I see in the bodies of movie stars. I wanted to change my bulging body into a more respectable figure, one that would make people admire me for my self-control.

Not all of us want to look like boys. But beneath our wish to tighten our flesh and flatten our curves, there may be a desire to enjoy the kind of authority, self-determination, and public respect that historically has been reserved for men.

Several years back, I came across an article in *Ladies Home Journal* that encouraged its readers to "Diet Like a Man." The article perfectly illustrated the long-standing link between masculinity, autonomy, and self-definition.[7] It suggested that the "will-power" required to lose weight is a quality more commonly found among men. The image accompanying the article depicted a woman dressed in a man's business suit attempting to tighten a belt around her oversized trousers. The obvious message being that a female body need not get in the way of a woman's pursuit of success and freedom, and that losing weight is an intelligent strategy for removing any remaining obstacles.

Unfortunately, there is some truth to the message in that article. The kind of power that comes from creating a "desirable" body can have many benefits, some of them professional. In our thin-obsessed culture, conforming to the slender ideal can help a woman secure a good job, a role in a play, TV show, or commercial, or a company promotion. It can help her compete in a world that is still primarily governed by men. How many women do you see in upper management in major corporations? How many of these women are large-framed?

One very successful—and attractive—woman, Katie Couric, reached the top of her profession by becoming anchor of the *CBS Evening News* in 2006. Despite her "normal" body size, the network's promotional department digitally altered her photo to make her appear slimmer. When Couric found out about the retouched version, she complained and quipped, "I liked the first picture better because there's more of me to love." She wanted to be judged by her abilities, not her dress size.

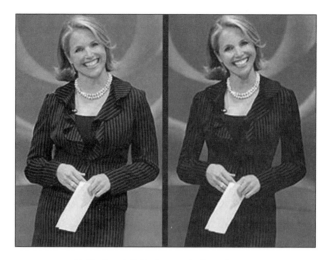

Katie Couric's before and after photos

The already superficial nature of media images is enhanced, in part, by their artificial production. The "perfection" of today's media models is created not only with the help of professional make-up artists, hair stylists, and clothing experts, but also electronically. This technology can lift a breast, tone a thigh, chisel a chin, and flatten a tummy with a click of the mouse. Even when we recognize these contrivances, we often feel helpless to ward off their influence. One woman explains:

> I know the pictures of the models I look up to are airbrushed and perfected with computer imaging. I know the cameras they use to photograph these women can make their legs look longer and their hips narrower. I know the models don't *really* look like that. But knowing this doesn't for a minute take away my desire to look just like them.

No matter how artificial and unrealistic these visual symbols may be, we still admire them. Appearance, not reality, reigns supreme. This is even true for political figures.

When Hillary Rodham Clinton first announced that she intended to run for a seat in the U.S. Senate, talk show host Larry King invited a panel of fashion experts on his show to comment on how the (then) First Lady could improve her looks. The day Clinton voted in the New

York primary, her office received numerous phone calls from constituents asking why the candidate had cut her hair. "The truth is that she'd just gotten up and wanted to be at the polls very early," Clinton's press secretary explained, "and so she just dashed out without blowing it dry. And the media focused on the 'haircut'—which wasn't."[8] In fact, hair has been one of Clinton's big issues throughout her career. When she went on *The Tyra Banks Show* during her 2008 campaign for the presidency, Banks spent several minutes going over various hairstyles Clinton had sported throughout her life, pointing out the merits of some and the pitfalls of others. A few months earlier the media's gaze wasn't on her hair but a little lower on her body. In July 2007, Clinton was spotted wearing a low-sitting, black, V-neck blouse while speaking on the Senate floor. Several days later, MSNBC devoted 23 minutes and 42 seconds to segments discussing Clinton's cleavage.

Even more recently, political commentators have been riveted by First Lady Michelle Obama's "sculpted biceps." While some praised this feature of her "well-disciplined body" as a "bracing symbol of American strength," others called for her to "cover up," insisting that "she should not be known for her physical presence."[9] Such rhetoric turns Ms. Obama's body into a public spectacle and puts her in a no-win situation: she must either downplay her "physical presence" in order to be taken seriously, or she must preoccupy herself with its upkeep because others seem set on defining her by it.

Regardless of your political disposition, it's easy to see how this emphasis is completely outrageous, frighteningly vacuous, and utterly hypocritical. Do Clinton or Obama's physical appearance really have anything to do with their performance and public service? Might the time spent debating Clinton's cleavage have been better used studying her position on major issues affecting the planet, like her foreign affairs policy, her response to global warming, or her stance on universal health care for Americans? Might the attention devoted to discussing Obama's biceps have been better directed at promoting some of the causes she cares about, such as education, veterans, homelessness, health, and the environment?

When Who You Are Is How You Look

The onslaught of media images teaches us to not only make judgments about celebrities, it also trains us to value everyone, including ourselves, according to physical appearance. Many of us become more invested in what we look like than who we are. We learn to see and experience ourselves as walking pictures and measure our beauty and goodness based on shallow facades. Depending on how much we allow mass-produced images to influence our self-perception, we may largely neglect our interior life and limit our self-reflection to the ruthless examinations we perform in front of the mirror.

This superficial way of seeing ourselves extends to our perception of others. The more we define and judge our worth based on appearance, the more likely we are to find ourselves doing the same to our friends, family members, co-workers, and people we don't even know! That is, we relate to the people around us based on their appearance rather than qualities that truly matter, like love, integrity, wisdom, and dreams.

This identification with how we look on the outside ultimately disconnects us from how our bodies feel on the inside. In fact, for many of us, experiencing our body *from within* may sound like a foreign concept. We might even be resistant to the idea of feeling—much less fully inhabiting—our bodies as they are. Some of us have had negative experiences, such as a serious illness or sexual trauma that make it difficult to feel comfortable in our flesh. But many of us simply don't like the way it feels when our bellies naturally expand as we breathe. We avoid the simple, physical satisfaction that comes from filling our stomachs with food, or we eat so much that we feel numb. We are afraid to feel too relaxed, because it might mean we haven't been working out enough. Or we shrug off the very thought of exercise because it would require us to be *in* our body. And what about the joy and sense of empowerment that comes from a physical connection to the earth? Many women don't even know such experiences exist.

Yet this physical body is the very ground of our existence. Why are we so eager to control, punish, and diminish it? Why do we resist and strive to eradicate the very flesh that connects us to the larger circle of life? Perhaps more to the point, how can we feel good *inside* our bodies if we experience them as little more than living pictures?

Moving Beyond the Image: Becoming Mindful of Your Body from Within

To practice peace with our bodies we need to learn how to relate to them as *more* than an image. We need to break through our fixation with how we look, embrace ourselves "as is," and delve into the deep and powerful experience of being in a physical form. By doing so, we end the cycle of female identification with appearance, create a mature appreciation of our bodies, and learn to enjoy what a gift our body can be. This can transmute our feelings of self-loathing into gratitude and respect for our bodies and the bodies around us.

To do this, it is useful to quiet your mind and turn your attention to your internal feelings and the energy that is pulsing through your body at this moment, animating your existence.

One exercise that I have found particularly helpful in this regard I call "Becoming Mindful of Your Body from Within." It is designed to refocus your attention on your inner experience, and it can help you reconnect with the feelings, energy, and sensations—the life—inside you.

Becoming Mindful of Your Body from Within

Start by quietly sitting or lying down and eliminating distractions that may keep you from focusing your attention on how your body feels from the inside. You can use the guidelines for sitting in Chapter 1, or simply find a quiet spot and bring your attention fully into the present moment by taking a few slow breaths.

As you do so, direct your awareness to your internal experience, more specifically, to your internal *physical* experience. How does your body feel at this moment? Can you sense it from within? Do you notice any pain, discomfort, or tension? Do you feel relaxed, anxious, tired, overwhelmed? Do you feel a sense of hunger or fullness?

Take your time. Often, our attention is so preoccupied with our external appearance that most of us are not accustomed to tuning into our "inner body."[10] So be patient with yourself as you do this practice.

To move your awareness deeper, I recommend doing a full body scan. Start by bringing your attention first to the feelings inside your feet, and slowly and progressively move your consciousness up the legs, through the stomach, back to the shoulders, and finally all the way through the head. If you have a hard time bringing your awareness to a particular part of your body, try tightening that part for several seconds and then quickly release it. This simple tighten-and-release technique can be used to cultivate awareness of different parts of your body and to enhance your ability to relax in your body.

What do you experience as you bring your attention to the various parts of your body? What is it like to be aware of your body from within, rather than focus your attention on the outside? Can you sense the subtle but vital energy field that pervades your entire physical form, animating every organ, cell, and limb? You may experience a tingling or buzzing, or some other sensation where your awareness is concentrated.

As you direct your consciousness toward your inner experience, try not to get caught in thoughts that may come up. Just *feel* without judging the feelings. As thoughts do come up (whether positive or negative) simply notice them without attaching to them. You might imagine writing them on a leaf and floating them down the river, as we did in Chapter 2. Throughout this process, keep bringing your attention back to experiencing your body from within.

If you get frustrated or distracted, or feel like you don't get it, don't worry. Learning to experience your body from within is a skill that develops with practice. Fortunately, you can do it almost any time and anywhere, not just when you're sitting or lying quietly. Whether you are stuck in traffic, sitting at your computer, or folding laundry, you can always shift your attention inward by taking a few mindful breaths and becoming present to your physical experience in that moment. With practice, this exercise will gradually shift your attention away from your external appearance, help you discern what your body really needs, and enable you to live more peacefully *in* your own flesh.

The Homogeny of Images and the Elitism They Create

It is not only the ubiquity of media images that impacts our relationship with our bodies and causes us to judge ourselves and those around us, it is also their homogeneity. In the visual landscape of popular culture, the physical form of the "flawless" female body varies in only the slightest degree. It is virtually shocking to see average-sized—much less full-bodied—women featured in advertising, mainstream magazines, or entertainment.

Because the bodies of "beautiful" women are so often depicted as young, tall, and slender, it becomes easy to believe that this is what true beauty looks like. And because this ideal dominates our culture's interpretation of beauty, it has become the norm—a norm that is *anything* but normal! Most runway models are about 5'11" tall and weigh less than 120 pounds, a body-type that represents about two percent of the female population. The average woman in the U.S. is roughly seven inches shorter and 35 pounds heavier than the industry ideal.[11]

The Religion of Thinness relies on the suppression of diversity. Alternative visions of beauty are excluded. Perhaps if we encountered glamorous likenesses of other body types more often, we would be able to embrace the slender bodies as just one possibility among many. But we are barraged with the slender archetype on such a repetitive basis that its cumulative effect erodes our capacity to choose. Men and women alike accept this limited vision of beauty as the only one because it is all most of us have ever known.

It's interesting to note that this suppression of diversity is rooted in the same kind of narrow-minded thinking that plagues certain factions within traditional religions. Such an exclusionary mentality assumes that there can only be One Truth and therefore only One Path to redemption. "Outside the church there is no salvation," is an early Christian example of this skewed perspective, which foreshadows the rigid, judgmental theologies of contemporary fundamentalists. While more prominent in some than others, samplings of this superiority complex are found in most religions. Even Buddhism, which generally has a great deal of appreciation for other faiths, has branches such as the Nichiren Shoshu sect that regards itself as "the One True Path of enlightenment."[12]

I am not suggesting that there is anything inherently wrong with a lean body. There isn't. Some females of all heights are naturally thin. But when the visual images of the women we encounter are uniformly slim, our capacity to see and value the beauty in bodies of all sizes and shapes is diminished. More and more, those of us who deviate from this unreasonable ideal are deemed unattractive. Fat people are frequently ridiculed or ostracized, and even those who are mildly overweight are considered undesirable or ugly.

It's tragic that so many women are willing to reject their natural bodies in pursuit of the fantasy worshipped by our culture. Conditioned by the same old images, we fail to see the beauty of the flesh we were born with as it changes in tandem with our life's transformations. Describing her feelings of inadequacy about her body, one woman recalled:

> I remember how my body looked *before* I had three children. I was young and fit and pretty back then. These days, it doesn't matter how much I exercise or how little I eat. I can't seem to lose weight and there's nothing I can do to make myself look better. I try not to look in the mirror anymore, because when I do all I see are my flabby arms, double chin, and ever-expanding midriff. It's depressing. Sometimes I really wonder how anyone could possibly find me attractive.

It's heartbreaking to think about how many women—including those who have just given birth (a sacred biological function)—suffer from similar thoughts and feelings and how much their beliefs about their bodies stifle their creative potential. When we believe there is only one way to be beautiful, we tend to scorn those features of our own bodies that make us unique: wide hips, small breasts, rounded belly, strong forearms, thick calves, double chin. Rather than appreciate the physical attributes that make us different from everyone else, many of us try to "fix" them, even to the point of submitting to cosmetic surgery. It seems that we would rather live in a world of Barbie dolls than accept and appreciate the beautiful variations of the female form as it is embodied from woman to woman.

This is an extremely exclusionary perspective, one that offers acceptance and "salvation" only to the "fittest." It creates a hierarchy in which the thin rise to the top, the fat sink to the bottom, and the "average" crave one extreme and fear the other. The homogenous Icons of Thinness establish a class of elite women and the rest of us are excluded from the heavenly kingdom.

The Elitism Embedded in The Religion of Thinness

The elitism embedded in The Religion of Thinness is perhaps most famously captured in the well-known quip attributed to Wallis Simpson, the Duchess of Windsor (1895–1986): "A woman can never be too rich or too thin."

However glib it may sound, her statement reflects the association between slenderness and social privilege promoted by media images. Many of the women that are put forth for our worship are simultaneously wealthy *and* slender. The curious connection between abundance and thinness often appears in magazine articles promoting "fitness." These articles presume readers have not only the time to renovate their bodies using the latest workout plan, but also the money to invest in the newest weight-loss products and exercise equipment.

To some extent, this link between thinness and affluence reflects social reality. Studies show that, on average, the higher a woman's household income, the lower her weight. Inversely, obesity is most prevalent among poor and minority women, especially African American, Hispanic, and First Nation women. Media reports of these trends rarely mention contributing social injustices.[13] Whereas rich people can afford a "thin lifestyle," which includes such luxuries as personal trainers, live-in chefs, weekly visits to the spa, and routine cosmetic surgery, people of modest means often can't even afford some of the basic requirements for good health, such as fresh, nutritious food, quality health care, and the time and a safe place to exercise.

Indeed, the association between wealth and thinness makes losing weight seem like a viable strategy for climbing the socioeconomic ladder. This is yet another way The Religion of Thinness seems to offer women a means to exercise power through the eradication of their flesh. For working and middle-class women, the desire to be thinner may be tangled up with the aspiration to enjoy the high-class lifestyles they see on TV or in magazines and movies. Several of the women interviewed by sociologist Becky Thompson for her multicultural study of eating problems traced their desire to be thin to a parental hope for greater economic prosperity. For those parents, "fat" was a sign of poverty. Immigrants to the U.S. felt that "fat" also signaled being un-American.[14]

The reality is that the fear of fat in our culture has both an ethnic and a socioeconomic bias. Contempt for fat people can function to disguise discriminations such as racism, classism, and sexism that have become somewhat less tolerated in the past few decades. If, as some people suggest, "fear of fat is a means of social control used against all women,"[15] it is a means that is used particularly against poor and minority women. Conversely, mass culture's glorification of thinness tacitly reinstates the privileges of those who are wealthy and white.

In recent decades, producers of media images have begun to cater to the diversity of real women by circulating depictions of women of color, maturity, or who could be interpreted as gay. We may appreciate the variety represented by such portrayals, but it's important to recognize that their true purpose is to broaden the commercial appeal of whatever is being sold.[16] These seemingly diverse images do not really call into question our society's racism, homophobia, economic disparity, or weight prejudice.

By glorifying a specialized and nearly unattainable body type this way, The Religion of Thinness has created unrealistic standards and subsequent suffering. A similar kind of elitism is evident in the history of some traditional religions, where select women are idealized and showcased at the expense of the majority.

The Virgin Mary is one of the most well-known examples of this dynamic. Mary's perfection is multifaceted: not only is she understood to be above the fleshly realm of sex and desire, but, according to Catholic doctrine, she was conceived without sin. (This teaching, established by Pope Pius IX in 1854, is commonly known as the *immaculate conception* and should not be confused with the "Virgin Birth" of her son, Jesus.) Like other holy women, her status was largely achieved through intense personal suffering and sacrifice. Throughout Christian history, church authorities went out of their way to emphasize and praise Mary's obedient response to the news that she would become the mother of the savior ("Let it be done unto me according to thy will"), turning her into an exemplar of female submission for other women to emulate. While Mary's image provided comfort and inspiration to countless female devotees, her privileged status did little to improve the overall plight of ordinary women, either in society or in religion.

The Illusory Power Elitism Offers

At first glance, submitting to The Religion of Thinness seems to make us more powerful. Many are motivated to lose weight by the promises of success represented by thinness: socioeconomic privilege, a competitive edge in a masculine world, praise and admiration, and other types of worldly rewards.

Unfortunately, our submission to this slender standard doesn't really make us stronger. It actually makes us *more subservient* to the dictates of popular culture. When we develop our potential and define our self-worth by sculpting and shrinking our figures, we are buying into the harmful myth that our female bodies—and therefore *we*—are inferior by nature, and that it is our job to attempt to improve or fix them. In her memoir, author Marya Hornbacher describes her anorexic-bulimic body as expressing "both an apology for being a woman and a twisted attempt to prove that a woman can be as good as a man."[17]

What we *really* need is not to be as thin as the women in the media or to prove that we are as good as men. We need to be the authors and artists of our own life stories, empowered to make our unique contribution to the world. We need to move beyond our idolatrous relationship with media images and create inspiring visions that speak to the beauty and diversity in all women.

Moving Beyond Our Idolatrous Relationship with Media Images

In the 8th and 9th centuries, a small congregation of Christians in the Byzantine Empire staunchly opposed the creation and use of images altogether. Motivated by a literal interpretation of the Ten Commandments that forbade the worship of "graven images," *iconoclasts* (people who oppose the veneration of religious images) feared that followers were becoming attached to the depictions of holy persons rather than the invisible truths they represented, and subsequently destroyed them. For that matter, Muslims and Jews have never allowed such depictions. Can you imagine our world without The Icons of Thinness?

We may not consciously worship popular culture's examples of womanhood, but many of us have an "idolatrous" relationship with its images. Moving beyond this relationship is a crucial step toward freeing us to love our bodies. This process begins with the practice of cultural criticism, observing the visual models we are encouraged to emulate and deconstructing both the messages they convey and our reactions to them. There are many ways to do this. We can:

- Develop our media literacy
- Critically scrutinize the media and ideals of female beauty with others
- Identify the ways visual ideals appeal to our insecurities
- Journal our responses to images we encounter
- Limit our exposure to mass media
- Deliberately collect the most extreme images we can find as a way of training ourselves to recognize their harmful lessons.
- Replace debilitating images with visions of womanhood that inspire us and foster a true sense of purpose

Developing Media Literacy

We can begin breaking our attachment to popular paragons of beauty by paying closer attention to the messages they carry. We need to become *mindful* of what we see. One way to do this is to practice a kind of cultural criticism called *media literacy*. Media literacy is the process of identifying, analyzing, and evaluating the messages conveyed in various forms of mass communications. We become "literate" in reading our culture's iconography of womanhood by asking questions like:

- Who produces the pictures and why?
- Who funds their production?
- What vision of "reality" do they construct?
- What biases and norms do they convey?
- Who benefits when we accept these biases and norms?
- What alternative representations are missing?

In addition to these questions about images specifically, there are a number of related, general questions that we can raise about The Religion of Thinness, such as:

- Why are the so-called "sexy" women in popular culture almost always thin?
- What stereotypes about large-bodied people do films, TV shows, and advertising perpetuate?
- How do media pictures implicitly teach us that we must be tall and thin to be healthy, happy, successful, and beautiful?
- Why do advertisements for "beauty" products assume there's something wrong with us?
- Who benefits when we buy into these assumptions?

Try doing this now. Look at the image of one of our modern-day female icons, Jennifer Aniston, on the cover of *GQ* magazine:

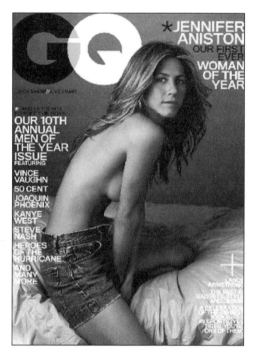

Cover of *GQ*, December 2005

There is no single correct way to analyze such an image. We all notice different things, depending on our previous experiences and expectations. One of the first things I see is that it appears on a magazine for *men*. This suggests, at least ostensibly, that the image is directed at male viewers. Like images of other models on magazine covers, its function is to sell the magazine by attracting potential readers. The assumption is that male readers will be attracted to a topless photo of Jennifer Aniston and will buy the magazine.

Yet I suspect that, as a woman, I'm not alone in being lured by the image, as well. Perhaps partly because the actress is virtually undressed and partly because she is so skinny, her image grabs the attention of both men and women. The messages are different for both genders, but they are also connected. For men: This is what a desirable woman looks like. For women: This is what you *should* look like if you want to be desired. Even the lines of her body—simultaneously smooth and yet firm—may spark different yearnings in her male and female viewers. For men: It would feel good to be next to this body, a yearning underscored by the fact that she is semi-nude and sitting on a bed, her breast is semi-exposed, and the single article of clothing she is wearing looks like it is so big it could fall right off. For women: It would feel good to *be* this body (and to have the power and confidence that comes with it).

Looking closely at the image, I notice the way her positioning on a bed without a shirt sexualizes her slender body, tapping into and reinforcing the association between slenderness and sexiness that most potential readers of this magazine already make, if only unconsciously. The combination of her curved-in, toned stomach (notice the space between her belly and her shorts and the shadow that at first glance makes her tummy look even thinner than it is) and her full breast (just enough is exposed to let us know it is ample) communicate an ideal body that is unattainable for most women without the "help" of surgery. Whether Aniston's body has been surgically "enhanced" is subject to speculation.

The fact that Aniston represents the pinnacle of *GQ*'s ideal of womanhood is evident in her status as the magazine's first ever "Woman of the Year," an honor she has been given in the "10th Annual Men of the Year" issue. This not only creates an ideal against which other women can be measured, it also connects Anniston's achievement of the "perfect" body with her success in a male-dominated world. Would it even be possible to bestow the honor of *GQ* "Woman of the Year" on a female who was not young, or thin, or "sexy"—a woman whose accomplishments had little to do with her physical appearance?

Who benefits when we buy into this fantasy of femininity? Who profits when this dream seems real? On an obvious level, of course, the answer is *GQ,* insofar as the photo on the cover lures consumers into buying the magazine. But all the other companies that advertise their products in the magazine benefit as well, and let's not forget all the other industries—beauty, weight-loss, fitness, fashion, cosmetic surgery, etc.—that profit indirectly when we absorb the messages communicated here.

This is just one example of how to critically analyze media images. However, it isn't the *only* way. I encourage you to come up with your own unique insights, because each of us sees these images through the lenses of our own life experiences (i.e., family history, ethnic background, social class, etc.). As you develop your critical skills, keep in mind that doing so will not make you immune to the manipulative power of the media, but the more you practice, the more you strengthen your resistance to this distortion by becoming an *active participant*, rather than a passive consumer, in your relationship with icons that glorify thinness.

We can further strengthen our media literacy skills by practicing with friends, family members, or co-workers who are similarly suspicious of The Religion of Thinness. The value of verbalizing your observations is apparent in this quote from a college woman who was struggling with anorexic tendencies:

> I was talking with my friend about the latest issue of *Cosmo* and how the models seem to be getting thinner by the day. We were both wondering why this is, when everyone knows eating disorders are a big problem. I was telling her how much I hate these images because they make me feel so unattractive. It was really validating because she just kept nodding and saying "I know what you mean." Talking to her helped me see how much I judge myself based on something so superficial.

Sharing our observations and critique with those we trust gives us the objectivity we need to see our feelings of inadequacy for what they are: conditioned responses to a toxic environment rather than a reflection of our true selves.

Write About the Feelings that Come Up

Some women find that keeping a journal is a helpful strategy for practicing non-judgmental observation, and this is another effective tool you can use for critiquing media images and becoming more mindful of their impact on you. For example, a woman who was working to overcome her pattern of yo-yo dieting started carrying a notebook in her purse to combat the dozens of advertisements she encountered on her daily subway commute. Each morning on her way to work, she recorded the internal dialogue that the billboards and wall posters with stick-thin models set in motion. Sometimes she wrote about the anxious feelings the images stirred, like "I'm afraid of gaining more weight," and "It feels like I'm losing control." Other times she wrote about the models, "She looks like she's about to fall over," "She's definitely skinny, but her eyes are empty and her smile is hollow," "She looks like she hasn't eaten in months." Giving voice to these feelings in her journal enabled her to reflect on them rather than be engulfed by them, and this in turn lead her to question whether such women really epitomized beauty.

One reason we idolize the ideal that tortures us is that the "perfection" it embodies seems to offer a cure for the larger fears and disappointments of our lives. Like many of the other false gods with which people struggle—money, sex, work, a relationship—The Icons of Thinness appeal to the part of us that feels unsatisfied or insecure, the part that is spiritually hungry. Journaling is a powerful tool both for increasing our awareness of emotional patterns that keep us stuck, and for developing an internal voice of resistance that allows us to "talk back" to messages that demean us.

Limit Your Exposure to the Media

Another way to diminish the effects of media images is to limit our exposure to them. The strategy here is to *intentionally* refrain from consuming mass-produced pictures for an extended period of time, whether it be for days or indefinitely. To the degree that it is feasible, we can choose not to watch TV, go to movies, read magazines, look at mail-order catalogues, or consume other forms of popular images. A recovering binge-eater who undertook such a "visual media fast" for six weeks described its effects:

At first I didn't notice much, except maybe how hard it was to not habitually turn on the TV. But after a few weeks, I found myself feeling more relaxed in my body, less focused on its "imperfections," and less judgmental of other women's "flaws." But the biggest lesson happened when I stopped my fast and started taking in the images again. It was a shock to my system, because suddenly I could see how totally plastic and artificial the women looked. I had not been really aware of this in the past, but they were much less appealing when I saw them in this new way.

Even a few weeks of giving up such images may help you see them in a different light, so that their contrived quality becomes more apparent and the perfection they seemingly embody no longer seems normal.

Collect Images and Critique Them

You can also go to the opposite end of the spectrum and *deliberately* collect media images that encourage women to define their worth through the contours of their bodies. Once you have some outrageous examples, critique them using the techniques previously mentioned. A few years ago, a group of college students undertook this proactive approach. They decided to make a giant collage of media images during Women's History Month to raise awareness about their damaging effects. Gathered in a dorm room late one night, they flipped through hundreds of pages of women's magazines in search of the *most* offensive pictures. This exercise took them out of their typical mode of consuming images as entertainment because it required them to pay close attention to their underlying messages. The next day, the students pasted the photographs they had collected on a wall in a well-trafficked area of campus. On top they wrote, "CONSIDER THE EFFECTS OF THESE IMAGES ON YOUR SELF-PERCEPTION." On the bottom, another sign invited students to respond to the collage by writing their own comments. A similar strategy that you can do by yourself is to collect magazine photos that embody messages of thinness and then ceremoniously rip them to shreds.

Even if you study pictures that idealize thinness more carefully, I still recommend limiting your exposure to them, because changing your perspective doesn't happen overnight. It is the product of persistent, deliberate re-training of your awareness. A woman who stopped buying women's magazines because, in her words, "they make me feel like hell," described her slow and steady progress:

> Even though I don't read the magazines anymore, I can't avoid seeing media pictures—they're everywhere. So as part of my recovery I've been training myself to *pay attention* to what these images are teaching me and to the feelings they bring up in me: jealousy, inadequacy, the desire for someone to adore me. It takes a lot of practice to *just notice* these feelings, rather than latch on to them, and I don't always succeed. But the more I practice, the better I get at it and the more I can channel my energy into developing my whole self and not just a thin body.

Remember, the wholeness we seek is not a state of perfection. Realizing our potential is an ongoing journey, rather than something we achieve once and for all. Discovering who we are is part of a larger spiritual process of learning to live more peacefully in our bodies, a process in which our searching is more important than our arriving. Zen teacher Katherine Thanas observes:

> It is wonderful to explore and continue turning over the question of 'who am I?' or 'what is this life?' so that we are simply open to what it means to be alive—to be in a body. And if we really don't know, which we don't, then the searching, the wandering, the questioning, the never-arriving, is a wonderfully liberating way to live.[18]

Every step you make away from your unhealthy obsession with thinness and toward a richer relationship with who you truly are is a vital part of your life's journey. Each of the strategies suggested here can help you take another step on the path of living more fully.

However, moving beyond the idolatry of thinness also requires us to find alternative icons to inspire our spiritual growth. One of the main reasons many of us became obsessed with The Icons of Thinness in the first place is that we didn't have healthier role models. But they are abundant.

Finding New Icons and Reinterpreting Old Ones

What icons might guide our journey by giving us role models worth emulating? What visible examples will encourage us to develop our talents and cultivate the truth, beauty, and goodness within us?[19] Ultimately, each of us must decide for ourselves what puts us in touch with our sacred values. What's important is that the icons we choose must go deeper than appearance. Most of us have encountered this different, ageless kind of beauty: in the wisdom that lines our grandmothers' faces, in the dimples of fat on a baby's legs, in the toothless smile of a child, in the scars on our bodies that remind us of both the risks we have taken and the vulnerabilities we continue to harbor.

As we search for images to orient our spirits, we must look to those that shatter the illusion created by The Icons of Thinness. Some women can find inspiration in religious icons.

Retrieving and Reinterpreting Images of Women in Religion

In recent decades feminist scholars have been retrieving and reinterpreting female heroines from traditional Western religions that inspire both spiritual growth and cultural critique. These alternative models of womanhood are empowering because they emphasize internal qualities, especially bravery, commitment, and ingenuity in the face of adversity.

Christian women may be surprised to learn of the power and courage of their spiritual foresisters. For instance, in the decades following Jesus' crucifixion, women supported the newly-forming Christian church both financially and by working as missionaries to spread the gospel. Archeological evidence suggests that some served as priests and even as bishops, while many assumed less official leadership roles in "house churches," private homes where Christians gathered for worship for more than two centuries following Jesus' death. Empowered by his message about the equality and dignity of all God's children, these women believed in their own spiritual authority. Many female followers no longer felt obliged to follow the dictates of man-made laws, whether religious or cultural. Liberated by faith, they refused subservient roles and, in so doing, provide us with an example of women's capacity to resist the social norms that stifle their spirits.[20] In fact, Biblical texts that order women to be silent and submissive are, indirectly, evidence of this self-confidence. As 1 Timothy 2: 11–12 declares: "Let the women learn in silence with all subjection. But I suffer not a woman to teach, nor to usurp authority over the man, but to be in silence." There would be no need to send women these messages if they were already quietly doing what they were told.

Within the Christian tradition, a number of scholars are re-envisioning the image of Mary. Instead of an icon of feminine obedience or a paragon of asexuality, they reinterpret her as a symbol of female strength. Mary not only suffered one of the most excruciating of all human experiences—the loss of a child—but she resisted the temptation to flee in the face of such suffering. She remained at the foot of the cross during the crucifixion until Jesus died, whereas most of the disciples had long since fled the scene. Also, in this new portrayal, Mary's virginity is not interpreted literally. Rather, it is seen as a symbol of her independence from the expectations of a society that fails to recognize her creative potential.[21]

This perspective of Mary finds visual expression in Our Lady of Guadalupe, the Hispanic representation of the Virgin that envisions her as an advocate for the oppressed. A number of *mujerista* (Hispanic feminists) have turned to her as a symbol of resistance to injustice as well as a source of affirmation of their ethnic identity and spiritual perseverance. Referring to the power she experiences from touching Guadalupe's image, a Mexican-American woman explains: "I feel that strength comes to me that keeps saying, 'Yolanda, you can do it, don't worry. I will always be here.'"[22]

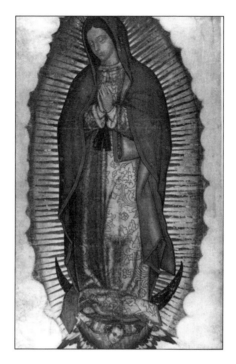

Our Lady of Guadalupe

Women of diverse cultural backgrounds are similarly discovering their inner strength through devotion to the Black Madonna. Paintings and statues of Mary holding the child Jesus that were originally created from black materials (such as ebony) or that turned black from natural causes (candle smoke, tarnish, etc.) survive from medieval Europe, an era when black symbolized fertility and regeneration.[23] In her book, *Longing for Darkness*, China Galland interprets the Black Madonna's darkness as a metaphor for wisdom and transformation. Together with other dark images of female divinity, the Black Madonna helped inspire Galland's journey out of addiction to alcohol into serenity and wholeness.[24]

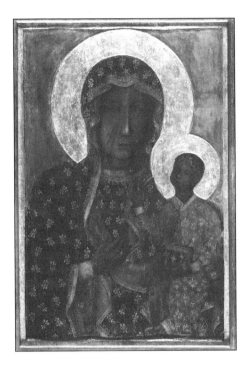

Black Madonna

The Virgin Mary is also held in high esteem within the Muslim tradition. She is the only woman the Qur'an mentions by name. Several verses in the Qur'an praise her, which inspired women to play a significant role in the development of early Islam. The Prophet Muhammad's first wife, Khadija Bint Khuwaylid, was the first person to believe in the truth of his teachings, and Aisha, another of his wives, was considered by her contemporaries to be an authority on Islamic laws. In fact, many women in this era were scholars and teachers, some of whom were frequently quoted by their male counterparts.[25]

A number of Muslim women today are drawn to the mystical tradition within Islam—Sufism—and find inspiration from the example of Rabi'a of Basra, a woman who is considered to be one of the greatest Sufi mystics of all time. She was born into poverty around 717 CE and later sold into slavery. Her owner is said to have freed her after observing her enveloped in radiant light while rapt in prayer. Upon her release, Rabi'a retreated to the desert where she chose a life of poverty, rejected numerous offers of marriage, and committed herself to prayer. She is perhaps best known for her unselfish love for God, which empowered her to resist external influences, as remarks attributed to her attest:[26]

> I am fully qualified to work as a doorkeeper for this reason: what is inside me I don't let out; what is outside me, I don't let in. If someone comes in, he goes right out again. He has nothing to do with me at all. I am a Doorkeeper of the Heart, not a lump of wet clay.[27]

Like their Muslim and Christian sisters, Jewish women may explore the resourcefulness and insight of women in the Torah. As Jewish scholar Judith Plaskow points out, the matriarchs of the book of Genesis are all strong, wise women who are independent-minded and fiercely concerned with their children's welfare. According to Plaskow, they also seem to have an intuitive knowledge of God's plans. Jewish women might also retrieve and re-interpret the legendary character of Lilith. According to Jewish folklore, Lilith was Adam's first wife and was mysteriously banished from Eden. In her reinterpretation of this rabbinic story, Plaskow suggests that Lilith was expelled by Adam because she insisted on being treated as an equal. In Plaskow's re-telling, Lilith represents the audacity we sometimes need to free ourselves from the expectations of others.[28]

Additionally, there are feminine manifestations of God in the Jewish tradition. Sophia is the personification of divine wisdom who breathes life into and cares for Creation. In the book of Proverbs, the figure of Wisdom accompanies God at Creation and commands all people to follow her ways.[29] The maternal quality of divine love in Judaism is expressed by the female figure of Shekhinah, who represents the indwelling presence of God. Although they are not visually expressed—according to the Jewish tradition—these feminine expressions of the divine are powerful sources of inspiration for Jewish women.

A number of images from Eastern religions are also possibilities for inspiring our spiritual growth. Similar to Sophia and Shekhinah, Shakti is a Hindu feminine manifestation of God, sometimes referred to as The Divine Mother. She represents the energy of life, the spirit found within all Creation. A multitude of other Hindu goddesses visually represent this energy, each embodying different aspects or qualities of the divine.[30] For example, Durga is often depicted as a beautiful warrior with a gentle face. Her 10 arms show her multifaceted and immense strength, some holding weapons designed to ward-off harmful forces. The tiger or lion she rides into battle is representative of her fierceness and her power in relation to the forces of nature. She is the benevolent but fearsome form of the divine, reminding us of the protective quality of God's power.

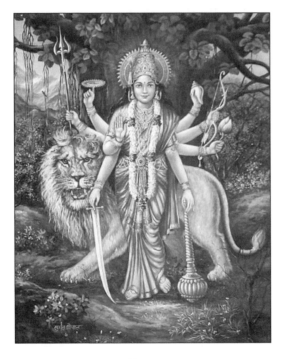

Durga

The Hindu goddess, Kali (also referred to as the "Dark Mother"), represents other aspects of the divine, particularly its creative and de-structive power. Her dark, four-armed body is usually dripping with blood, her neck is ringed with a garland of skulls, her waist sports a skirt made of human arms, her eyes are bulging, and her tongue is protruding between her teeth! In some depictions, Kali holds a cleaver, a severed head, and a flower in three separate hands, while the fourth gestures not to be afraid. Although her formidable image may shock Westerners, she represents life at its fullest: deadly and fertile.[31] Her image is a prime example of how sacred symbols can encourage us to own and integrate the various aspects of ourselves. This integration is crucial for our development as whole—rather than perfect—persons.

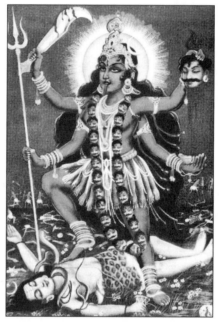

Kali

Kuan Yin (a.k.a. Guan Yin or Guanyin), the Buddhist *bodhisattva* of compassion, represents the beauty and strength that is already in us. As a fully-enlightened being, Kuan Yin, who chose to forgo nirvana in order to save others, is the embodiment of kindness. She is also known as "She Who Hears the Cries of the World." Kuan Yin perceives the sufferings of all sentient beings and takes whatever form is necessary to help them. She can bring fearlessness to those who are frightened or in danger, and peace to those who are agitated and worried. Many Buddhists believe that concentrating on her image not only brings comfort to those who are burdened, but also inspires those who suffer to seek healing by helping others.[32]

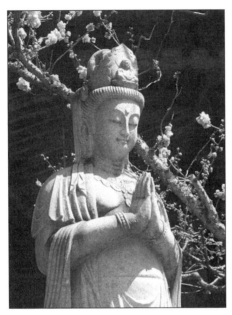

Kuan Yin

These are but a few of the female icons from traditional religions that represent something far more meaningful than the ideal body: love, compassion, integrity, bravery, commitment, wisdom, audacity, and even ferocity. Their images teach us something about the beautiful dance of life and death and the power of suffering that has been transformed. In so doing, they call us back to our true inner purpose, awakening us in various ways to the life that is around and within us.

Other Feminine Symbols of the Sacred

"The Goddess" is an ancient symbol of feminine sacred power. In contrast to the traditional Western view of God as an old man with a long, flowing beard, female images of the divine affirm the female body in its diverse shapes and colors and throughout the various stages of life. Because of its natural changes and cycles, including its capacity to give birth, the female body is an appropriate symbol for the life-giving power of the divine.[33] As mentioned early in this chapter, one prominent depiction of the Goddess, Venus of Willendorf, emphasizes her role as the giver of life, The Great Earth Mother. Her huge breasts, wide hips, enormous thighs, and protruding belly remind us of women's creative potential. Such images were once revered and may help some of us reconnect with the power inherent in our own bodies—the same power that The Icons of Thinness encourage us to domesticate, diminish, and disconnect.

For most of her devotees, the Goddess is not a being who is out there but a *symbol* of the fundamental power of life and death, the natural energy that ebbs and flows throughout creation and in our own flesh. In this worldview, the earth itself is imagined to be the Goddess's body, with its people, animals, plants, and minerals all belonging to the great "web of life" that is created and nurtured by the power of the Goddess.[34] This view reminds us that our own bodies are sacred and the energy that flows through us is part of the same force that gives life to all things.

Precisely because women have a long-standing association with physicality, images of the Goddess have the metaphoric potential to break our attachment to thinking of our size or shape as "never good enough." By representing divine power in the likeness of women, such images affirm the strength and beauty within us—both spiritual and physical. A woman who was recovering from years of compulsive eating explains:

> I used to think of God as a supreme male being—a kind of giant, though invisible, father figure in the sky. It took me a while to realize that this image was cutting me off from my own spiritual potential as a woman. Now I think of God—or Goddess—as a loving power within myself. She encourages me when I want to give up. She nurtures me when I'm down. She's there for me when I'm scared and lonely. She's happy for me when something good happens. The more I listen to her, the less I obsess about my body and the less I worry about what other people think.

Whether we envision what is sacred as male or female—or both or neither—we need to find images that encourage us to love and nurture our bodies and spirits. The more we devote our attention to these empowering images, the less we will find ourselves chasing after hollow fantasies of thinness.

The Inspirational Power of Contemporary Women

In addition to female images of divine power, contemporary women who dedicate their lives to helping alleviate the pain of others can be great role models. For example, you may admire the African American author, poet, feminist, and human rights activist Alice Walker, whose work includes contesting the practice of female genital mutilation in parts of Africa. Or you might look up to Eve Ensler, the Jewish American playwright and activist who wrote *The Vagina Monologues* (1996) and *The Good Body* (2004), and who has made it her mission to end violence against women, including the violence we do to ourselves by hating our bodies. Winona LaDuke, the Native American activist and author, founded the Land Recovery Project to enable native peoples to reconnect with sacred Mother Earth by buying back land that was taken from them. Jean Kilbourne is a cultural critic whose insightful documentaries, books, and lectures have taught thousands of women to see through the lies of advertising images. These are but a few of the extraordinary and inspiring women who are working to create a better world by challenging the legacies of oppression, prejudice, and violence that humans have been struggling with for far too long.

But it is not only these "accomplished" women who are worthy of emulation. There are sources of inspiration much closer to home. For many of us, female relatives, friends, coworkers, and teachers demonstrate models of love, compassion, strength, and wisdom. A woman who struggled for years with body hatred found it helpful to tape photos of her mother and grandmother on the side of her bathroom mirror.

> Each morning I look at them when I'm getting ready. Their short, plump bodies remind me of how ridiculous it is to think that my body would ever conform to the tall, slender ideal. It's just not in my genes, and I'm tired of wasting my energy wishing

it would be. What I also notice when I see their pictures is the warmth of their smiles and the pain in their eyes. I know they have given more love than I can imagine and suffered things I'll never know about.

Whatever the details of their lives, and regardless of their size, the generosity of these everyday heroines can provide an inspiring example when our lives feel small and aimless. If we give them attention, our relationships with real women who support our growth *as whole persons* can replace a devotion to airbrushed idols who are anything but real to us.

None of these images—whether they are portrayals of goddesses or portraits of our grandmothers—will magically enable us to love our bodies or make peace with food. Their healing power comes from their capacity to make us mindful of our deepest values and what truly matters. A recovering anorexic-bulimic woman explains:

> If someone were to ask me who or what I wanted to be, I used to point to examples of famous actresses, because they seemed to have everything you could possibly want, especially their bodies. In the course of my recovery these past few years, I've discovered new images of what it means to be a woman. Women like Joan of Arc and Mother Theresa remind me of the courage and kindness that I want people to remember me for. Do I really care if, when I'm dead, people say, "Wow, wasn't she thin"?

The Calling to Be Real

The empowering potential of these spiritual, historical, and contemporary female role models underscores the impoverishment of the superficial images to which so many of us are devoted. By contrast, the alternative images offered in this chapter challenge us to develop ourselves in all our complexity and diversity. These alternatives are far from exhaustive. They represent just a fraction of the possibilities that might spark our imaginations, encourage us to explore the larger meaning of our lives, and enable us to live more peacefully in our bodies. Such visions call us not to be perfect, but to be real.

4

FROM CONTROL TO CONNECTION

"The Rituals of Thinness" and Our Need for Transformation

Sophia's knee was killing her, but she had at least two more miles to go. It looked as though it was about to snow. She tried to distract herself from the pain and cold by going over the number of calories she had eaten that day. "200 for breakfast," she began. "Not bad for a Saturday morning," she assured herself between breaths. "500 for lunch...or maybe it was closer to 550? And did I include the mints? I'll round it up to 600 just to be safe." Having eaten nearly 800 calories already, Sophia knew she would have to be careful at dinner. That's where she frequently got into "trouble." "At least today is a long-run day," she reminded herself. "800 calories in, 800 burned," she figured, recalling the charts she'd memorized from a fitness magazine. "Now if I can only keep it to 400 calories or less at dinner...." Sophia's thoughts turned to her parents, who were coming to visit. She hadn't seen them since her divorce, and she knew they'd be impressed by her weight loss.

Life is change. One moment slips into the next, and as the tide of time flows onward, our lives are altered. Sometimes these shifts take the form of major life passages, like finishing school, losing a loved one, having a baby, or getting married. But change also happens in more ordinary and subtle ways, as our aging bodies attest. Experiencing these shifting tides can be scary, because they make us aware of just how little control we actually have. Rather than go with the flow, many of us try to steer our tiny ship with ever more determination. In an effort to deal with the insecurity, stress, loss, and uncertainty that change so often leaves in its wake, we reach for ways to feel more in control.

One of the most common strategies our culture provides for "taking charge" is to focus on our bodies, particularly through the use of weight-loss rituals, such as counting calories and carbohydrates, having daily weigh-ins, separating the "good" foods from the "bad," and running the treadmill. *The Rituals of Thinness* offer a myriad of ways to cope with life's impermanence. But, our weight-loss rituals do more than just give us a way to feel more on top of things; they also keep us connected to the ultimate purpose of thinness. In the same ways that The Icons of Thinness are the visual reminders, The Rituals of Thinness are the everyday practices through which we recommit ourselves to this goal. The repetition of these pursuits reinforces the message of The Myth of Thinness and plants it deep inside our body, so that its supposed truths feel like second nature and our efforts to reduce our bodies become habitual, even automatic, and, in some cases, compulsory.

As a result, many of us become trapped by the very rituals we perform to free ourselves from feelings of insecurity and distress. Instead of giving us a sense of mastery, our weight-loss disciplines start to master us. If we don't do them, we feel off-kilter. If we don't eat the "right" foods, if we don't exercise "enough," if the scale shows that we weigh more than we think we should, if we don't double-check ourselves in the mirror, our whole life can feel out of balance.

When this happens, our capacity to evolve through change is stifled, and our lives tend to feel stuck or stagnant. Externally we might look cheerful and productive, but inwardly we feel depressed and numb. We find ourselves going through the motions—in relation to food and exercise and in our lives as a whole—instead of actively engaging with the challenges we encounter and using them to learn and grow.

What we really need is not to be in control of our lives but to feel capable of handling whatever situation comes our way. We need a sense of *stability* amid this endless flux—an inner strength that comes from being grounded. The Rituals of Thinness cannot give us this foundation. They are a ruse.

In this chapter, I explore the connection between The Rituals of Thinness and our desire for control. We will discover how rituals function and have the power to "get under our skin." I will show how our weight-control practices recycle an antiquated view of the body and fuel the war we wage against ourselves. And we will find new ways to practice peace with our bodies through mindfulness.

How Rituals Function and the Needs They Serve

Rituals are symbolic actions performed in a formulaic and repetitious manner that help us move through the big and small changes of our lives by providing a sense of stability. They can be as formal as a traditional wedding ceremony or as ordinary as a handshake. Consider some of the most commonplace rituals in our culture: watching TV sports on Sunday, going to the annual New Year's Eve party, enjoying a cup of coffee in the morning, brushing your teeth before going to bed. Each of these customs guides us through transitions—from weekend to workweek, from one year to the next, from sleeping to waking, and back to sleeping again. Not unlike their more formal religious counterparts, these informal rituals give us a sense of order that allows us to move through, rather than get lost in, the endless changes of our lives.

In *religious* contexts, rituals have various functions depending on the setting. I want to focus on three common aspects of ritual in many conventional religions that also play an important role in The Religion of Thinness.

1. The *repetitious* nature of ritual gives participants a predictable course of action to rely on and trains their

spirits to stay centered on an ultimate purpose. Religious examples abound. No matter where they are or what they are doing, devout Muslims take time to pray five times a day, each time preceded by obligatory cleansings that prepare them to give honor to God. Hindus regularly serve the divine through a practice called *puja*—devotion to images of beloved deities, which they honor with food, flowers, incense, song, and other symbolic gestures of reverence. Buddhists practice meditation seated in a lotus position, quietly watching their breathing. Jews observe the Sabbath with prayers over candles, *challah*, and wine. These activities create a reliable, habitual pattern by which devotees can find order in their lives. Participants know when, how, and where to perform them, and this consistency and repetition has a stabilizing effect.

2. **The *symbolic* nature of ritual reflects and reinforces the ultimate purpose that is embraced by the religion and its adherents.** Rituals are not just routine actions. They are behaviors that have *symbolic* meanings, and each time adherents engage in one, they are taking a moment out of their daily lives to remember what is most important. Symbolically, ritual gestures, movements, and recitations recommit those who perform them to their sacred values. Muslims kneel in prayer with their foreheads touching the floor to express their total submission to God. Buddhists sit with an erect and motionless posture to cultivate and express a still but alert presence of mind. Christians who participate in the Eucharist receive the body and blood of their savior (whether metaphorically or mystically) in their own bodies—a gesture that recalls and celebrates the life, death, and resurrection of Christ. Eating the communion wafer will not satisfy their bodily hunger, it is a way to nourish them spiritually.

3. **The *embodied* nature of rituals allows the ultimate purpose they symbolize to "get under our skin."** Ritual practices are the most *physical* aspect of religious traditions. By enlisting our senses through corporeal activities—eating, drinking, singing, touching, smelling, bowing, posturing—rituals connect our minds and our bodies, creating a kind of "muscle memory" of the truths they aim to foster. It is the embodied quality of ritual practices that enables them to permeate a very deep level of our being—beyond our conscious awareness—making them highly resistant to change.

When rituals function in a healthy, positive way, these three aspects are extremely empowering. The *repetitive, symbolic, embodied* nature of ritual gives us a solid foundation on which to build our lives. The predictability of ritual behavior allows us to relax and let go even though we never really know what new circumstances life may bring. The symbolic character of our ritual actions grounds us in the truths we hold dear, which empowers us to deal with difficult situations and feelings. When our ultimate purpose gets under our skin, we can operate confidently from our core values and move forward amidst change with hope and courage.

But ritual can have a destructive side, as well. In fact, the very aspects of ritual that make it so powerful can also corrupt it, turning it into a means for control instead of stability and connection. That is what happens when we practice the rituals of The Religion of Thinness.

The Use of Ritual in The Religion of Thinness

The Religion of Thinness prescribes a set of rituals for its adherents just as all religions do. The activities we are expected to engage in are relatively specific, they happen at regular intervals, and they reflect the three principles just outlined. We may practice one or more of them, depending on the degree and kind of obsession with food and thinness with which we struggle. Our most common Rituals of Thinness include:

- Counting calories, carbohydrates, and/or fat grams (before, during, and/or after eating)
- Weighing ourselves on the scale
- Calculating body fat
- Measuring waist size
- Exercising compulsively and to extremes
- Planning and carrying out a binge
- Purging
- Dieting
- Obsessive eating behaviors
- Checking ourselves in the mirror
- Comparing ourselves to our culture's idea of a "good" body
- Berating ourselves when we don't measure up

The problem with these food and body rituals is not their repetitive, symbolic, or embodied qualities—the three features that give traditional religious rituals so much power. The problem is that the ultimate purpose they reinforce is not our *true purpose*, and the security that thinness promises is an illusion.

When Behaviors Become Ritualistic

Any behaviors become *ritualistic*—mechanical, compulsory, and empty—when we are disconnected from our ultimate purpose. Our prayers can become automatic or even selfish. Meditation can be used as a form of escape. Even everyday rituals can become mindless activities when our hearts are not engaged.

The Rituals of Thinness are particularly prone to becoming ritualistic because they do not reflect our fundamental values in the first place.

Instead of promoting our health and recommitting us to the qualities in life that we truly cherish, like love, compassion, courage, and wisdom, they keep our attention fixated on the tenets of The Religion of Thinness.

For most of us, our involvement begins when we engage in seemingly innocent behavior. You may have started counting calories, monitoring your appetite, and exercising regularly in a genuine effort to be *more healthy*. One young woman describes the well-intended beginnings of her eating disorder:

> I was in high school and had several friends who wanted to lose about 10 or 15 pounds—though now that I think of it, none of us were really overweight. We all started dieting and exercising and I was pretty good at it. I started to get hooked on the compliments and gained confidence. Losing weight made me feel in control for the first time. So I intensified my efforts until it got to the point where if I ate anything that normal people ate, like a sandwich or spaghetti, I'd spend several hours burning off the calories.

Good intentions can blind us from seeing the extent to which our efforts at self-improvement can function as a form of self-destruction, particularly when their primary aim is not peace of mind, body, and spirit, but thinness.

Exercise is a prime example. Various studies suggest that young women exercise more for appearance (i.e., thinness) than for reasons of health.[1] One study found that 95 percent of female respondents said their primary motivation for exercising was weight-loss.[2] Often, the preoccupation with burning calories removes any potential pleasure or satisfaction that comes from staying fit. For many women, exercise either becomes a burden and they quit, or they develop unhealthy compulsions around it. However, when women exercise to improve their fitness, to relieve stress, and even to cope with psychological trauma, it can be a life-affirming way to connect with the body.

Popular articles that encourage fitness reinforce the link between exercise and thinness, and turn ordinary activities—such as walking—

into symbolic rituals that recommit us to The Religion of Thinness. The article from *Fitness* magazine shown below is a good example of this. Here you are told you can "walk off your weight." That sounds like a very good idea. Even if you don't try the fat-blasting, bun-chiseling, treadmill workout this article recommends, you have to walk some-time. Why not use the process of getting from here to there to serve the ultimate purpose of thinness? However, when we connect an activity as ordinary as walking to this goal, we see the world through a distorted lens and become more deeply tied to the weight-loss mentality.

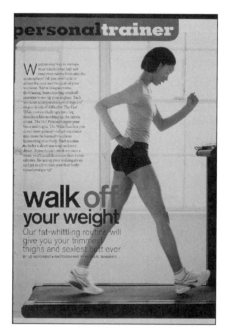

"Walk off Your Weight" – *Fitness*, January 2001

The slippery slope from healthy to harmful exercise illustrates how difficult it is to recognize the insidious nature of The Rituals of Thin-ness. Many of us are not aware when our well-meaning effort to "get in shape" turns into a method to "get in control." We may not realize how easily our attempts to eat in a more healthy way can become obsessive patterns of consuming only certain foods or counting every calorie we ingest. It is extremely difficult to recognize that many of our various efforts to monitor, measure, and contain our figures simply reinvest our bodies and spirits in the tenets of The Religion of Thinness.

This religion grips us on a very deep level precisely because we incorporate its myths and ideals into our very flesh through our repetitive actions. Just as religious practitioners engage in rituals sanctioned by their tradition, so we honor and embrace the ultimate purpose of The Religion of Thinness through our body-controlling disciplines. As a result, our weight-control efforts plant the belief that thinness will "save" us—that somehow it will make everything okay—deeply in the soil of our flesh and spirit, making it very difficult to uproot, *even when we know, at some level, that it's not true.*

What's most insidious about weight-loss rituals is that they distort two of the body's most basic needs: eating and movement. Once you've bought into The Religion of Thinness, it becomes very difficult to engage in—much less enjoy—these natural functions without feeling compelled to use them as an opportunity to further your "progress" on the road to a better body. Eventually, it becomes all but impossible to perform even the most innocent of actions, like eating breakfast or going for a walk, without tying them to the goal of thinness.

Even if you are aware that your exercise and eating patterns are harmful or obsessive, you may not be able to stop them. This is not because there is something wrong with you. Their repetitious, symbolic, and embodied qualities make them extremely compelling, if not compulsory, especially when other areas of your life seem to be spiraling out of control. A woman who began exercising excessively as a way of dealing with her mother's cancer describes the progression of what she called an addiction:

> I used to run several miles every evening both to keep my weight down and to unwind from the stress at work. But when I learned of my mother's illness, this healthy habit became an addiction. I not only needed to run every day—missing a day made me feel crazy—but I needed to run farther and farther just to feel okay. Part of me couldn't fathom giving up running any more than I could fathom living without my mother. So I had no interest in stopping.

Our unhealthy rituals may masquerade as their more helpful counterparts, but they not only fail to provide the inner strength we need to handle adversity, they often leave us feeling more desperate than ever to get back in control.

The Rituals of Thinness and the Quest for Control

Control is at the heart of The Religion of Thinness. Its rituals aim to provide a sense of security, safety, and familiarity. The way women talk about their bodies and food illustrates this association. One working mother who was raising three children and trying to save her second marriage expressed the connection in the following way:

> When I feel anxious about the chaos in my life, I find that dieting gives me a sense of order. Being thin makes me feel like I'm in control. It fills a void and helps me cope, at least for a while.

This sentiment is similarly expressed in the comments of a college student who struggled with periodic episodes of bulimia:

> I see other girls who are thin and I hate them. Well, I don't really *hate* them. I envy them, because they possess exactly what I most want but don't have: self-control.

Weight-loss rituals appeal to us not just because they give us the feeling of taking charge, but also because slenderness itself is seen as representing the epitome of control. In our image-driven culture, a woman's tightly-contoured body announces to the world that she is disciplined and free, that she's "got it together." Not surprisingly, many of us imagine that having such a body would automatically give us the confidence and power we feel is missing in the rest of our life.

It is no coincidence that many of us were first initiated into The Religion of Thinness as we entered adolescence, a time when our bodies felt "out of control." Dieting is one of the few rites of passage our culture provides girls on the threshold of womanhood. The physical and emotional shifts that accompany puberty—from menstruation to mood swings—demand attention. Girls usually gain weight at this stage of life, which is nature's way of preparing for the possibility of childbearing—a fact of which many are unaware. Yet instead of getting taught how to honor this process and navigate it in a healthy way, young women feel pressure to engage in various body-altering remedies and rituals; and, many begin even before adolescence. One study of 4th grade girls revealed that 80 percent had already dieted![3] Regardless of when we were introduced to The Rituals of Thinness, many of us use them well beyond puberty—through pregnancy, motherhood, menopause, and into old age—to defy our body's transformation into a more mature female figure.

Control and the Pregnant Body

Whether a woman feels joy, ambivalence, or distress upon discovering that she is pregnant, these emotions are frequently layered with some level of anxiety about the changes taking place in her body. If she herself is not worried about gaining too much weight, it is likely that others will sound the alarm. Pregnant women are constantly reminded—by well-meaning doctors, family members, friends, co-workers, relatives, and even complete strangers—of this horrible danger. Never mind that putting on weight during pregnancy is a natural part of the process, essential for the health of both baby and mother. Forget that the increased hunger most pregnant women experience—usually after the first trimester and throughout lactation if they are nursing—is the body's way of ensuring that it has enough nutrients to both feed the newborn and give the mother stamina. For many women, the fear of gaining weight and losing control clouds the entire experience of childbearing.

The pregnant female body has not always been viewed as a threat to women's self-control. There was a time in history when this form was celebrated and honored rather than feared, not in spite of, but because of, the powers of fertility it so obviously displayed. Again, recall the Venus of Willendorf in Chapter 3. This small statuette of a fully-rounded female body reveals the reverence some ancient cultures had for woman's creative powers. If you stop to think about it, this attitude of reverence makes a lot of sense. After all, the pregnant body is where life is conceived, nurtured, and birthed into the world. It is a living, breathing symbol of the mystery and miracle of creation. No wonder some ancient cultures understood the power of God in feminine terms!

If you have experienced anxiety about gaining weight during pregnancy, please don't berate yourself for it. Like so many others, you have been conditioned to feel this way by a culture that worships fat-free bellies, boyish hips, and sag-free breasts. Interestingly, it is precisely the parts of the female body that represent fertility that we are most encouraged to manipulate, control, or diminish through various Rituals of Thinness. Little wonder that, instead of feeling reverence and pride over our pregnant and postpartum girth, many of us end up feeling embarrassed or ashamed.

Even if we want to celebrate our body's natural expansion during pregnancy, we still must deal with the societal pressure to stay fit (i.e., thin). The growing fascination with celebrity pregnancies during the past decade has made this mandate all the more imperative. The vast majority of the attention received by pregnant movie stars revolves around their seemingly superhuman ability to stay sleek and slim throughout and after their pregnancy. The message is clear: your child-bearing body can be a source of pride, as long as its weight gain is confined to your belly and breasts. However, this propaganda flies in the face of logic and obvious health risks. For example, women with eating disorders commonly experience complications of pregnancy, including higher rates of miscarriage, morning sickness, preterm delivery, and cesarean section. Fetal complications include premature births, growth retardation, low birth weights, smaller head circumferences, and low Apgar scores.[4]

Even if you happen to use good sense—or lack the "will-power" to stay slender while pregnant—don't worry. Entire magazines are dedicated to the task of keeping you "fit." Let's practice some cultural criticism by studying this cover of *Fit Pregnancy*:

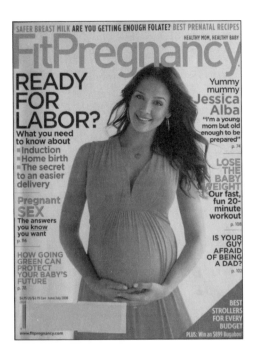

Fit Pregnancy, June/July 2008

Here is a magazine that purports to be a resource for holistic, prenatal, health information. Articles informing you about home birth, safe breast milk, being ready for labor, creating a green environment for your child, and issues fathers face during pregnancy indicate at least some commitment to promoting a woman's overall well-being in the course of those nine months.

However, the magazine clearly conveys the message that appearance matters when you're pregnant. You want to stay sexy—a "yummy mummy." And to make sure you haven't forgotten The Rituals of Thinness, *Fit Pregnancy* will help you "Lose the Baby Weight" with its "Fast, Fun 20-Minute Workout."

This mentality is pervasive. When I was pregnant with my first child, I attended a class sponsored by a well-known hospital corporation to learn about breastfeeding. The first thing the instructors did was hand out a brochure that listed 10 benefits of nursing your child. At the top of the list, trumping all the others and in the number one spot: *Breastfeeding helps you lose your pregnancy weight faster.* Apparently, losing your pregnancy weight is even more important than the health benefits, economic advantages, and bonding opportunities of breastfeeding.

What does it say about our society when losing weight is a higher priority than the health of our children? What kind of cultural mindset judges pregnant women according to how many pounds they gain before giving birth, and how many they take off once the baby is born?

This is a culture obsessed with control.

The "Burden of the Flesh" in Western Culture: Plato and the Christian Legacy

Since the early days of Western civilization, the body has often been viewed as an obstacle to the pursuit of truth, goodness, and freedom; and, denying the flesh has been considered spiritually virtuous. The concept dates back to ancient times and is perhaps best illustrated in the writings of the 4th century BCE Greek philosopher, Plato, who saw the body as a "prison" from which our souls long for release. In his view, the body interferes with the pursuit of wisdom: its sensations, vulnerabilities, cravings, and pleasures lead the soul astray. Plato believed that a person attains knowledge and truth only by "despising the body and avoiding it, and endeavoring to become independent of it."[5]

These ideas significantly influenced Christian beliefs about the role of the flesh in the search for salvation. Although early Christian theologians rejected the Platonic view of the body as a prison, they nevertheless saw it as a potential barrier or distraction on the path to spiritual virtue. We find this in the letters of the Christian apostle, Paul, (died c. 67 CE), who writes in his second letter to the people of Corinth, "…while we are at home in the body we are away from the Lord." (2 Corinthians 5:6). Though biblical scholars debate Paul's intention in such texts, early church fathers interpreted his ideas to support their mistrust of physicality. Jerome (died c. 420 CE), the highly influential Christian apologist, spoke of the "burden of the flesh" and warned monks to wrap their hands in their robes when exchanging the sign of peace, lest the touch of a woman incite their lust and lead to sin.[6]

The idea of flesh as a burden led to ritual observances meant to torment and tame the body so that the spirit could be freed. This connection between self-inflicted suffering and salvation is apparent in the ascetic practices of early and medieval Christians, who denied their physical cravings and sometimes deliberately mortified their bodies (wearing hair shirts or heavy chains, or flagellating themselves) as a method for cultivating holiness. Christian ascetics were thought of as "spiritual athletes" who trained and disciplined their flesh to achieve a higher state of purity. By renouncing earthly pleasures such as eating certain foods, drinking wine, engaging in sexual activity, and even sleeping, ascetics sought to reorient their worldly (physical) desires toward an other-worldly (spiritual) purpose.

The popular contempt for the body revealed in some aspects of Christian theology and ascetic practices is ironic given this religion's more official teachings about the inherent goodness of the body.[7] The Christian doctrine of the Incarnation—the belief that divinity became flesh in the person of Christ—affirms the intermingling of body and spirit. The gospels suggest that Jesus celebrated and was concerned about physical life: healing the sick and eating with "sinners" were central to his ministry. Many of his parables focus on food. The central symbol for Jesus' message of God's reign was the image of a great feast to which everyone was invited. Christians today continue the practice of bringing their bodies and spirits together by sharing in the rite of Communion. Unfortunately, within this tradition, the anti-body aspects of Christianity have tended to overshadow the more affirming views.

Mind over Body

During the past 400 years, Christianity's predominant view of the body as inferior and untrustworthy became increasingly secularized. In the 17th century, this view gained new momentum with the writings of the French philosopher, René Descartes. He identified the essence of human beings as their capacity to reason: "I think, therefore I am." Descartes saw the mind and body as completely separate entities, with the mind (or "self") in the seat of command. Like a military commander overseeing troops, the Cartesian self—the "I"—orders the body around, monitoring its every move, disciplining its every desire.[8]

Many of us inherited the belief that our appetites are tied to a dangerously wild force within us that, when left alone, threatens to overtake or destroy us completely. We believe the body is either a "temple" or a "tomb," depending on our ability to control its cravings, especially the urge to eat. "How I feel about my body depends on how well I've stuck to my diet," a compulsive dieter explains.

> On days when I'm in control and don't stray from my food plan, I feel a sense of accomplishment and pride. But whenever I veer off course in the slightest degree, I can see every piece of flab and bulge on my body, and I feel disgusted. When this happens, I do whatever I can to turn things around—hours at the gym, laxatives, fasting, you name it—whatever it takes to get back in control.

Without realizing it, too many women practice a kind of asceticism similar to some historical Christians. We deprive or discipline our bodies to "redeem" ourselves, to make us more acceptable and worthy—if not in the eyes of God, then in the eyes of others. Through our Rituals of Thinness, we affirm that control is holy and suffering is redemptive—as if our growling stomachs somehow make us better people, superior to those who "can't restrain their appetites" and who shamelessly enjoy the pleasure of eating. Ultimately, we become engaged in a battle of control over our bodies, and inadvertently turn rituals into weapons.

At War with Our Bodies: When Control Turns to Violence

Feeling in control gives us a sense of power over something that must obey our will, whether it's an unpleasant feeling, an insatiable appetite, or an unruly part of our body. Control is also the form of power that is engaged in warfare, where the aim is to use destructive tactics to conquer, and ultimately destroy, an enemy—such as fat. In the words of spiritual author Starhawk, control is essentially "power-over." It is the power of the bomb, the power of the gun.[9] Control produces relationships of estrangement, where one person—or thing or idea—is pitted over and against the other. Ignoring and denying the physical signals our body gives us that it needs attention, such as hunger or pain, reflects this combative attitude.

This militancy is embedded in The Rituals of Thinness. Though we turn to such rituals for empowerment, what they are actually asking us to do is to destroy ourselves. Our desire for control can blind us to the violence they encourage us to inflict on our bodies and spirits. Consider the language used in the weight-loss industry. Women are told to "burn off fat" as if they could light a match to it and see the flames. Advertising and magazine headlines call for "Triumph in the Battle of the Bulge," or "Win the War against Obesity." These are angry phrases that connote violence and hatred. Are these the feelings we want to have about our bodies?

The concept of burning off fat leads us to another popular Ritual of Thinness: popping weight loss pills.

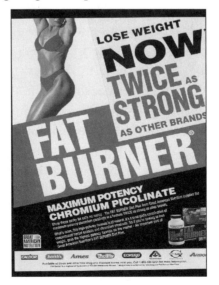

Magazine advertisement for "Fat Burner"

This advertisement is for a product called "Fat Burner." It is one of a multitude of weight loss supplements available during the past several decades. Nowadays, a Google search for this term produces about two and a half million hits. A common marketing approach is to promise users that they do not need to exercise, can eat whatever they like, and can even "sleep away pounds." Here, "Fat Burner" boldly brags that it is "twice as strong as other brands," an unsubstantiated boast, while the smaller print admonishes, "Show those pesky fat cells no mercy." This ad treats fat as if it were a kind of demon to be exorcised. The language itself encourages a violent attitude towards our bodies: *Show no mercy.* It sounds like a line from the Medieval Inquisition! We are supposed to "burn" our fat cells, torch them like heretics at the stake!

Despite this, there is little evidence of the efficacy or safety of this product's "all natural" ingredient, chromium picolinate.[10] In fact, this mineral has potentially significant negative effects on health. One study shows that it is more likely to cause DNA damage and mutation than other forms of chromium.[11] In mice, the consumption of this chemical results in skeletal defects in their progeny.[12] In fruit flies it causes chromosomal aberrations, impedes development of offspring, and can lead to sterility and lethal mutations.[13] And a review done by the Committee on Mutagenicity at the UK Joint Food Standards and Safety Group found several cases where it was connected to renal failure (a condition in which the kidneys stop working and the body's ability to eliminate waste is either inhibited or destroyed).[14] Encouraging women to take these pills is another destructive act against them.

Of course, the ad is highlighted by a shapely, well-toned female figure in an eye-catching, red (in the original) bikini. Notice how only a portion of her body is displayed. This is a recurring tactic in ads that use the female physique to sell products, one that not only reinforces the focus on women's bodies, but also has an element of violence. In these kinds of ads, the woman is fragmented, dismembered, objectified, lifeless.

Just as we aren't surprised to see a picture of only the torso of a sexualized woman, it doesn't come as much of a shock that bold, red letters promise that this "high potency" product is "twice as strong as other brands." After all, we want **strong** supplements, just as we want a **strong** body and a **strong** mind, so that we can "stay in control" and defeat the enemy, our body.

What does it say about our culture's values when companies are allowed to peddle unsafe chemicals to "help" us create a particular body size and shape? What does it say about our culture's attitude towards our bodies when we are encouraged to wage war not just on our fat cells, but on our entire organism?

For centuries now, our culture has been steeped in the belief that the flesh inhibits the progress of the spirit, and that therefore we must combat and conquer our carnal nature. This notion is embedded in our collective consciousness. It is part of our cultural legacy, our inherited worldview, and our collective dysfunction. Most us of have been conditioned to believe that our body holds the key to our happiness, and that thinness is the physical symbol of this sanctified state. Every time we practice The Rituals of Thinness, this conditioning gets etched a little bit deeper into our minds, bodies, hearts, and spirits, until it feels like it has always been there and thus becomes increasingly difficult to notice, much less challenge or undo.

The Problem with Control as a Strategy for Coping with Change

One of the problems with battling our bodies is that often the "enemy" proves to be quite stubborn. Many of us have experienced how hard it is to stick to a diet, and how depressing it feels when we fail yet again. Control is an unreliable method for containing such a persistent force. Ironically, the intractable nature of our opponent leads some of us to compulsively engage in weight-reduction rituals for years, even decades. What's more, in trying to control an adversary that ultimately can't be defeated, many of us become caught in the paradox of ascetic behavior: our effort to deny the body ties us ever more tightly to it.[15] This paradox is familiar to anyone who has tried to restrict her eating.

Dieting entails a repression of physical needs—to eat less than your body wants. But the hunger you experience from denying your cravings draws your attention back to your body. Interestingly, the sensation of hunger itself is an important part of this process: it is a signal that you are making "progress." It can also be a frustrating reminder of the limits of your dominion over your physical needs. In the end, denying your appetite makes you *more*—not less—attached to it. We are caught in a prison of food and weight-related thoughts, feelings, and behaviors. A bulimic woman in her thirties recalled how the insidious cycle began for her in what seemed like an innocuous attempt to lose a few pounds:

> I was feeling sort of lost after college. All my friends seemed to know what they wanted. Of course, all of them were happy and thin. I wasn't. I needed to gain some sense of control. Losing weight became the answer, and the sense of accomplishment was so satisfying after I lost an initial 10 pounds, I intensified my efforts.
>
> Gradually, I became totally absorbed in my own little world of food and calories. I kept notes of every calorie I ingested and burned. Nothing else seemed to matter. Eventually, my efforts to whittle down my body backfired and I became bulimic. Now every night, it's the same routine: lock myself in the bathroom after dinner, turn on the water, bend over the toilet…. What started as an attempt to manage my body has made my life totally unmanageable.

Whether or not you suffer from bulimia, elements of this woman's struggle likely reflect your own. Even small attempts to change our rituals demonstrate the strength of habit and the elusive quality of control. We may resolve to stop skipping meals or to never binge again, but we've forgotten how to eat in moderation. We may vow to stop thinking we're too fat, yet still cringe when we see ourselves in the mirror. We tell ourselves, "I'll just have a salad for dinner," only to find ourselves raiding the fridge at midnight. We say, "I'll go to the gym three times every week," and never get there.

The list of promises made and promises broken is long. The harder we try to regulate our eating, the more futile it seems and the more desperate we feel. The more we long to transcend our appetites, the more we find that our attitude toward food is far from carefree. This is because the whole idea that we can master our body—that we can rise above its fluxes and cravings, that we can defy the inevitable pull of gravity and the process of aging, that we can win this war against our carnal nature—is a fantasy.

In fact, I believe this war against our flesh conceals a desire to *connect* with our bodies, to spiritually evolve *through* their waxing and waning. On some level, we yearn to get back in touch with what it feels like to live *in* a body—hungry, full, tired, pumped, peaceful, sexy and every other experience available! And, some wise part of us knows that this connection is *fundamental* to the sense of empowerment we seek.

Practicing Peace with Our Bodies

If what we really want is to connect with and experience our bodies more fully, why do we go to war with them? One key reason is that The Rituals of Thinness intensify our somatic experience. Starving, bingeing, and purging are all *physical* activities that make us hyperaware of our bodies—even as they make us more estranged from them. Tragically, many of us rebel against our bodies because it is the only way we know how to stay connected to them.

There is another way to live. Feeling at home in your flesh is a much more empowering experience than fighting it. Imagine how calm you'd feel *without* the conflict that comes from constantly trying to control your weight. Instead of judging, measuring, obsessing, and feeling inadequate, you would enjoy and appreciate the natural uniqueness of your body. You would experience health, energy, and the pleasures of eating and moving instead! Perhaps this is what we have unconsciously been attempting to do all along—reconnect with the physical ground of our being.

After all, we are physical creatures. It is through our tangible, sensing, feeling forms that we experience every single thing that ever happens to us. We need to connect with our bodies—live *in* them—not conquer them. Practicing peace with our bodies is what fosters this connection and returns us to our inner wisdom, the real source of our strength.

If rituals are embodied actions that symbolically link us to our ultimate purpose, then we need to go within. There we can discover what matters most to us and create meaningful new rituals, both symbolic and practical, to honor and move peacefully through the transformations of our bodies and our lives.

Developing New Rituals to Nourish Body and Spirit

Right now there is a stranger in your midst. Although you may not yet be able to sense its presence, this stranger is a fundamental part of you. It is the physical body you live in, the one you have been battling and tormenting for so long. Now, you have an opportunity to call a truce, get reacquainted, and become friends.

The kinds of rituals that can nurture this growing friendship are embodied practices that promote *transformation, not domination.* They involve discipline, to be sure, but not the kind that is punishing or destructive. In contrast to control, which is so often a knee-jerk reaction to fear or pain, this kind of discipline entails conscious intention, presence, and commitment, as well as effort, guidance, and perseverance. Embodied practices don't repress or oppose desire. Rather, they teach us to be present to our passions and to find healthy outlets for them. Unlike The Rituals of Thinness, which teach us to respond to our problems by policing our bodies, practices that integrate our bodies and spirits:

- *(re)train* us to stay calm when the anxiety of change overwhelms us

- cultivate courage when we feel frightened or helpless

- help us to observe our cravings when they get insistent

- make us feel grateful for food that is nourishing and delicious

- energize our minds and bodies and help us concentrate on the moment

- *(re)connect* us to the values and ideals we hold most dear

The world's religions abound with examples. The dietary laws of the ancient Hebrews fostered awareness of the sanctity of life while solidifying their identity as a people and distinguishing them from the cultures around them. The Buddhist emphasis on mindfulness not only deepens the enjoyment one experiences from eating, but it also invites practitioners to consider how the food they consume connects them to the rest of the world, including the various groups of people who grew, harvested, sold, and prepared it. The Islamic observance of *Ramadan* not only unifies Muslims across the globe, it also creates empathy for those who are hungry, while reinforcing surrender to God.

Of course, each of these examples involves the consumption of food. But notice what is different in these rituals compared to The Rituals of Thinness. For one thing, they do not focus on personal gain and are not invested in helping devotees improve their figures. Muslims do not fast during Ramadan to get skinny. Jews do not observe kosher dietary practices because eating these foods promises to make them attractive in the eyes of others. Buddhists do not eat mindfully as a way of getting control of their lives. Instead these rituals reconnect people to their bodies, to their communities, and to their most sacred values. Such observances symbolically affirm and express commitments that are far more likely to enrich lives than those of The Rituals of Thinness.

Spiritual practices that help us heal our relationship to food and our appetites engage *both* our bodies *and* spirits in the process of self-transformation. Their aim is not to conquer or transcend our physical cravings, but to discover that we can love all aspects of our humanity, including our flesh. With patient repetition, our new rituals can teach us how to ground ourselves in the present moment and connect us to what we most value. Then, from this place of strength, it becomes possible to let go of our control agendas and evolve through life's changes instead of trying to resist them.

Practicing peace with our bodies requires us to develop or seek out spiritual disciplines that are suited to our individual personality and our particular path. The rituals we choose may vary as much as the sizes and shapes of our bodies. In the remainder of this chapter, I offer a few suggestions for rituals that engage our physicality in the process of spiritual growth.

Embodied Prayer

Whether you gravitate toward conventional religion or alternative spiritual resources, the practice of prayer in its many manifestations offers a way to intentionally and ritualistically use your body as an expression of what you value most. Prayer strengthens us by connecting us with the deep truths of our lives, those that nourish us and give our lives meaning.

Many of us have been conditioned to think of prayer as something that takes place in our minds or solely through words. For some, prayer is about quietly folding our hands and asking God for help, or expressing our gratitude toward "Him." Though embodied prayer often does involve some expression of gratitude, it isn't restricted to mental or verbal affirmations, and it doesn't have to involve a "higher power." Embodied prayer comes in many forms, any of which can be celebrations of what we value, or ways of giving thanks for the gifts we have been given. Or they can be activities designed to help us calm our minds and center ourselves on what is most true for us.

Embodied prayer is not new and, when considered in this sense, is not restricted to dialogues with God. Kneeling, bowing, singing, clasping hands, sitting quietly, raising our arms, or closing our eyes are all age-old physical expressions associated with prayer. When we engage in this type of prayer, our bodies serve as vehicles for expressing our hearts' intentions. Those intentions are deeply personal and unique to each individual. They can range from learning to accept our reality without resistance to getting involved in social movements that challenge the status quo. When Jewish theologian Abraham Joshua Heschel was asked to describe what it was like to march in Alabama with Dr. Martin Luther King, Jr., he responded, "My feet were praying."[16]

Intentionally using our bodies to communicate what is important to us through prayer brings our physical and spiritual dimensions together. It is the awareness we bring to the physical act that makes it powerful and tranformative. The simple act of bowing or kneeling can be done mindlessly because we are "supposed" to do it, or it can be done consciously to express humility, gratitude, and respect. Sitting quietly with our eyes closed can be a way of dissociating ourselves from the outside world, or it can convey our desire to be more present to the here and now.

When we attentively engage our body in a search for inner wisdom and strength, the results can be truly transformative. A woman recovering from years of anorexia nervosa and bulimia found what a vital role her body could play in her healing. She created a practice of mindfully scanning her body. As she moved her consciousness through her body, she envisioned it as a vessel of healing and service:

> I usually begin with my hands and feet, bringing my attention to my toes and fingers and working my way in and around the various parts of my body. I identify my inner organs, my lungs, heart, stomach, and so forth, as well as my eyes, nose, mouth, and ears, and I offer these parts of myself to God, so that my body becomes an instrument of peace for myself and others. I do this before I get out of bed in the morning. It only takes a minute or two, but it makes a huge difference in how I feel throughout the day.

Whether or not we are religious in the traditional sense of the word, we can practice engaging our bodies to re-focus our spirits when we feel our energies pulled back to our obsessions with weight and eating. There are many ways to do this:

- Mindfully walking, using each step as a way to ground ourselves in our bodies and in the present moment or to help us let go of destructive thoughts and emotions

- Using symbolic objects to stabilize our attention, like lighting a candle to center ourselves when we're feeling scattered, or burning incense to create a sacred atmosphere and help us become aware of our breathing

- Simply bowing our heads, holding our hands together, and giving thanks before a meal

- Eating in silence (alone or with others) to help us enjoy and stay mindful of the food we consume

- Singing or playing or listening to our favorite music

As these examples suggest, virtually anything you do with or for your body can become a ritual act of care and transformation if you do it with loving attention.

Below is a mindfulness exercise that I like to use as a form of embodied prayer.

The Power of Life in Your Body

Start by taking a comfortable position as you did in the exercise called "Becoming Mindful of Your Body from Within" in Chapter 3. Do the body scan outlined there and bring your attention to your inner sensations, how your body feels from the inside. Specifically, try to get in touch with the energy you feel inside your body at this moment, the humming life within you. Take your time. If you don't feel it immediately, sit patiently and continue to gently direct your consciousness inward, keeping it focused below your neck. If thoughts or feelings come up, simply observe them and let them go. Focus on the physical sensation of the energy within. Just be present to it. Try to feel it. And do this for at least five minutes.

Once you connect with this feeling (and even if you don't), take a moment to notice that this energy is the same one that permeates the world around you. The creative force flowing throughout your body is the same one that enlivens the birds chirping outside your window, the trees growing in your back yard, the wind blowing through their branches. It gives life to the sun and breathes through the motion of the waves and the tides of the sea. It makes the seed grow and the baby be born. It is this evolving power that drives all transformations, from the changing seasons to the shifting contours of your body as it ages. It is the life force—*chi* in Chinese philosophy—and you are connected to it. It is both beyond you and within you. The physical form you live in—your body—is a uniquely beautiful manifestation of it. In this very moment, the life force in your body is connected with the life force in every other living creature, with all creation. You have the capacity to experience this because you live in this body. Be mindful of that truth.

After a few moments of resting in this awareness, you might contemplate the following questions:

- If you could harness the life force that flows inside your body and direct that energy in the service of anything, *what causes would you choose?* Personal happiness? World peace? Your family's well-being? Political issues? Saving the environment?

- *In what way would you serve these causes?* Would you march in the streets like King and Heschel? Would you spend more time with your children? Take long walks in the woods? Ride your bike to work? Volunteer on behalf of those who are socially or economically disadvantaged? Go back to school? Take more time for sitting quietly in prayer and meditation?

When you're finished reflecting on these questions, gently bring yourself back, but take this feeling of deep connection with you. Let it strengthen and empower you, especially when you're feeling anxious or unsure. Use it to deal with whatever you face from day to day using the grace that is already within you.

The beauty of this exercise is that it helps us understand, on an experiential level, that there is more than one kind of power. The "power-over" you have sought and cultivated through The Rituals of Thinness operates on the principle of control. But there is another kind of power, what Starhawk calls the "power-from-within,"[17] which is the inner strength you feel when your thoughts and actions are aligned with your true purpose. It's not that you can control what happens, but that you are capable of dealing with whatever happens because you feel a connection to something much bigger than your personal existence.

You may want to take a moment to let yourself feel the natural gratitude that comes up as you realize the truth of this connection, knowing that whatever challenges you face, you can find your way back to this basic wisdom by tuning into the power of life inside your body. In fact, this gratitude is an acknowledgement of the inherent abundance of life—a recognition that "there is enough," indeed, that "I am enough," which runs counter to the doctrine of scarcity enshrined in The Religion of Thinness. This insight can transform feelings of emptiness into feelings of fullness in both body and spirit.

The ordinariness of most of life's blessings makes them easy to neglect. Practicing embodied prayer helps us cultivate the gratitude we need to enjoy and appreciate these everyday gifts. Many of us have bodies that are still relatively healthy, despite all the torture we've put them through. Most of us have access to clean water and nourishing, tasty food. A lot of us have families that love us, however imperfectly. Each of us has our own list of blessings for which we can give thanks. Whatever our condition in life, when our mind starts racing with thoughts about food or thinness, we can stop what we're doing, straighten our posture, relax our chest, bring ourselves into the present, contemplate that which we truly value, connect to the life force within us, and be thankful for *this* moment. Practiced repeatedly, this simple form of embodied prayer can transform our compulsive energy into a more peaceful attitude of gratitude—a calm, abiding awareness that we already have everything we need to be whole.

The Path of Yoga

A growing number of people are practicing yoga as a means for reconnecting with their bodies. The term *yoga* (literally, "to yoke") has a double meaning. It means *uniting*, as in yoking together, as well as *training*, as in bringing under the yoke. Yoga is a spiritual discipline that helps unite the body, mind, and spirit through the holding of various physical poses, or *asanas,* and through conscious breathing.

Though yoga is a traditional Hindu practice, the path of yoga is open to persons from all spiritual walks of life; it doesn't require any image of God or set of beliefs. Because of its long history—over 2000 years—and vast and diverse community of practitioners, yoga means different things to those who practice it. Some people do yoga to maintain or increase flexibility, to give their minds a rest, or to cultivate both physical and spiritual health. Others consider it a pathway for uniting with a higher power.

Many women with eating problems have found that the breathing and meditation exercises of yoga, along with the *asanas*, are effective ways to redirect their attention away from their external appearance to how their bodies feel from the inside. The poses are metaphors for our lives—they express the desire to bring harmony to the various parts of ourselves. The emphasis is not on how a pose looks, but on how it teaches us to feel both the strength and freedom that emerge when the parts of our body are aligned with each other. Yoga's breathing exercises are designed to cultivate similar feelings of connectedness. Breath is a bridge between our bodies and minds. As such, it is a powerful tool for calming our spirits. When we find ourselves fixated on food and thinness, breathing consciously, slowly, and deeply can change the energy of our craving by moving our attention back to our internal experience of our bodies and returning us to the present moment.

Christina Sell, a former body builder and fitness professional, writes about the essential role yoga played in her recovery from an eating disorder:

> For much of my life, exercise was one of my strongest weapons in the war with my body. By over-exercising, refusing to rest appropriately, and obsessing about my shortcomings…I perpetuated [this] war.

For Sell, the practice of yoga became a way to integrate her deepest values with a physical regime, which transformed her relationship with her body. She examines this experience in the following passage from her book, *Yoga from the Inside Out:*[18]

> If my intention is to offer peace, and my understanding is that yoga can lift some of the veils that block me from experiencing the ever-present reality of grace, then to practice with harsh criticism and violence is truly out of spiritual alignment. To practice yoga with spiritual alignment requires me to soften, to relax, and to listen to my body with compassion and sensitivity.

You can find the larger story of Sell's transformation in the same book. She passes on the compassion she's developed for herself and others by teaching and practicing yoga today.

Exercising to Gain Energy and Strength, Not to Lose Weight

As you seek ways to love and appreciate your body, you will likely need to change your approach to exercise, especially if you have used it as a form of punishment or avoided it altogether. Learning to enjoy physical activity that gets your heart beating requires a shift in outlook. Instead of seeing exercise as a road to thinness, we can focus on the ways it makes us stronger, increases our energy, relieves stress, and promotes general well-being. When it is not tethered to the goal of losing weight, pursuing fitness can be a source of integration and healing, a way to practice peace with our bodies.

The belief that a fit body has to be thin is so commonly accepted in our culture that few would dare to question it. However, hundreds of studies indicate that thinner is *not* necessarily healthier. In 2005, for example, the Center for Disease Control reported on a major study that found people who were underweight had an increased risk of death. That same year, another study found that being underweight poses increasing health risks as one ages.[19] More recently, a 2008 study of more than 5,400 adults found that half of overweight people and one-third of obese people are "metabolically healthy," meaning that they had healthy levels of cholesterol, blood pressure, blood glucose, and other risks for heart disease. The study also showed that about 25 percent of people who fall into the "healthy" weight range actually had at least two cardiovascular risk factors that are usually associated with obesity.[20]

There's a big difference between fitness and thinness. It's possible to be fat and fit or thin and unhealthy. Body size and shape are *not* indicators of metabolic health.

Any sedentary person can become more active, regardless of their size or weight, which opens the door for all of us to enjoy physical activity and take advantage of the healing it can bring. In *Great Shape: The First Fitness Guide for Large Women*, Pat Lyons and Debora Burgard offer an abundance of suggestions and encouragement for large-bodied women who want to discover the joy of exercise.[21] Lyons and Burgard are leaders of a movement called Health at *Every* Size, which promotes fitness for people of all shapes and abilities through physical activities that are suited to their bodies. *Curves* fitness centers, which tend to be more welcoming to large-bodied women than most other commercial gyms, is one of the fastest growing franchises in America.[22]

Exercising for energy and strength can take multiple forms, and the key is to find activities you enjoy. If you are not inclined to working out at the gym, you might join an athletic team, practice tai chi, play tennis, or go golfing, hiking, dancing, or rollerblading. You need only observe the natural tendency of children to run, jump, skip, and play to understand your body's need to be physically active. This need does not disappear as we grow older and spend less time at the playground, and our spirits suffer if we ignore it. Whatever you do, try not to think about burning calories. Simply take pleasure from moving and being in your body.

A recovering bulimic woman in her 30s described the changing role of exercise in her healing process:

> For most of my life, exercise was all about losing weight. I'd calculate the amount of physical activity I needed to burn the calories I ate. Now that I'm in recovery, I still find myself craving that good feeling you get from physical exertion, but I try to find ways to exercise that don't feel like I'm punishing myself. Instead of spending three hours a day strapped to an exercise machine at the gym, eyes glued to the calorie monitor, I take a

long, leisurely bike ride on the path along the river. Or I go for a walk in the early morning, clearing my head before I start the day. The point now is to enjoy the experience of being *in* my body, instead of pushing myself till it hurts.

Enjoying our bodies depends on *knowing their limits.* Those of us with a history of exercising compulsively can cultivate this knowledge by paying attention to the physical cues our bodies give us. Exercise does not have to be taxing to be effective. Anything from mowing the grass to going for a walk can give you a way of processing the thoughts and emotions that you have habitually buried with food and the drive for thinness. Instead of adhering to old time or distance requirements we've established for ourselves, we can practice being flexible by slowing down and taking a break when we start to feel tired or achy. If we're worn out from running, for example, we might shorten the distance, slow our pace, or try walking instead. These are acts of kindness towards our bodies that can replace the habit of pushing them beyond their limits. The point is to find forms of movement that harmonize with our actual physical needs, rather than exhaust ourselves. Practicing peace with our bodies means finding a balance between the activity and the rest we need.

While for some of us exercise can be addicting, others find it nearly impossible to get moving. This is not because we are "weak-willed" or "lazy." Exercise resistance is a complex problem and there are many reasons to feel unmotivated. Traumatic experiences that involved our bodies, including unwanted sexual experiences, can impair our connection to the energy that moves us. Many of us grew up with social or familial messages that reinforced an inactive lifestyle. Some of us who enjoyed playful activity when we were younger lost interest when it became focused on competition. Whatever our physical history, identifying the impact of such experiences is a vital part of re-inhabiting our flesh. Healing psychological blocks to exercise opens us up to the possibility of enjoying our bodies as we move in ways that make them stronger.[23]

The spiritual disciplines outlined here—embodied prayer, yoga, and exercising for energy and strength—are just a few possible ways to foster a more loving connection to your body. There are numerous other ways you can deepen your friendship with your flesh. Developing self-care rituals suited to your particular pleasures and needs equips you to handle the uncomfortable emotions that contributed to your eating problems. When you're feeling anxious or depressed, you can soothe yourself by taking a bath with essential oils or by massaging your feet and hands with your favorite lotion. Some of us have access to more formal self-care rituals. Instead of throwing our money at the latest weight-loss gimmick, we can spend a day at a spa that emphasizes overall health (as opposed to thinness), or visit a massage therapist who specializes in holistic healing. We might also pursue complementary forms of medicine for some of our health care needs. Medical traditions such as acupuncture and *Ayurveda* address the whole person—body, mind, and spirit—in the process of healing. The point is to simply find whatever resources are available to you that will help you transform your adversarial relationship to your body. Change your paradigm from control to connection. As you do this, you will begin to experience the feelings of confidence and security you sought in the first place.

Practice, Practice, Practice

Whatever embodied practice you choose to do, the key is to *do* it. Don't wait for some idealized time in the future when you are "ready." Change starts today. The perfect moment—the *only* moment—is *now*. If this sounds intimidating, please remember that the goal isn't getting to a place where you'll never have to struggle with food again and where you'll be blissfully happy with your body. That's the same kind of control agenda that got you to where you are today. The key is to find new, life-affirming, body-loving rituals that work for you, and do them. Practice, practice, practice. The more time you spend focused on learning to live peacefully in your body—rather than trying to transcend or control it— the more new patterns of muscle memories you will plant, and the more new patterns of thinking and acting will gradually take root.

Changes are often two steps forward and one step back. At first, going in a different direction might feel uncomfortable, or even wrong. A backlash of feelings—fear, depression, and confusion among them—may surface when you stop harassing and chastising your body, and you may resort to old, unhealthy habits. A woman in recovery explains:

> When you get to a new point in healing, going back is familiar. Even when you know it is bad, it is familiar. That is a really lonely place in your growth. You get to a place in healing, in spiritual growth, where you recognize these patterns...you don't want to go back, but that is what is familiar.[24]

Even a misstep on the path to recovery can be an opportunity for growth. Your supposed failures actually make your spiritual practice, whatever form it takes, all the more valuable and necessary. When you find yourself eating more than you want, when you feel reluctant to eat what you need, or when you hear those old tapes playing in your head, slow down, breathe deeply, and return to your new practices that ground you in your physical and spiritual center. Through repeated effort, you can cultivate the wisdom and courage you need to transform your "setbacks" into learning experiences.

It is encouraging to remember that wholeness is not a state of perfection but an ability to be present to the challenges and changes of life *as it is*. Each day we make numerous choices, either to relate to life directly with the support of our spiritual resources, or to continue trying to avoid life by controlling our bodies. Healing is a matter of changing both our consciousness and life habits. Author Anne Lamott reflects on her recovery from bulimia, expressing the transformation that comes from years of practicing a spiritual program:

> When I feel fattest and flabbiest and most repulsive, I try to remember that gravity speaks; also, that no one needs that plastic-body perfection from women of age and substance. Also that I do not live in my thighs or in my droopy butt. I live in joy and motion and cover-ups. I live in the nourishment of food and the sun and the warmth of people who love me.... It is, finally, so wonderful to have learned to eat, to taste

and love what slips down my throat, padding me, filling me up, that I'm not uncomfortable calling it a small miracle.... Whatever it was, learning to eat was about learning to live—and deciding to live; and it is one of the most radical things I have ever done.[25]

If we want to change our relationship to food and our bodies and learn how to flow with change instead of going to war with it, we need to practice new rituals that connect us to our deepest values. We must respect our bodies in ways that nourish our spirits. And, as we shall discover in the next chapter, we must also practice taking responsibility for our own well-being and the welfare of those around us by enlarging our moral perspective.

5

FROM JUDGMENT TO RESPONSIBILITY

"The Morality of Thinness" and Our Need for Virtue

Maya stood in line at Starbucks waiting to place her order. As often happened, she'd planned to get up early to finish some work and hadn't had time for breakfast. She really wanted yogurt, a banana, and a scone with coffee. But she remembered a magazine article she had read about the hidden calories in foods that most people assume are healthy. "Like scones and yogurt," Maya thought to herself. "Better go with the banana and coffee. Even better—just coffee."

Standing there, she wondered whether it was possible for her to go the whole morning on just a cup of coffee. She had several important meetings scheduled. Would she be able to concentrate? The challenge was inviting, and the purity of it was enticing.

Finally it was her turn to order. "You know, I think I'll be really good *today," Maya told the stranger across the counter. "Just give me a large coffee. Leave room for skim milk!" she rushed to add as she dug in her purse. "That's all, thanks."*

Everyday we make an endless number of decisions. Some are routine, like whether to have yogurt and a scone with our coffee. Others are more complex, such as: *Where should I invest my energy? How should I respond to people who hurt me? How can I pursue my own interests and dreams while caring for the needs of others?*

We may not always be aware of it, but we're making decisions about how to live and who to be every moment of every day. While it's true that our freedom to choose one way or another may be limited by any number of forces beyond our control, it is never totally eclipsed. Like it or not, we always have options. And when we operate from a strong moral center, we make choices that bring harmony to both ourselves and the world. Such a place is essential to our spiritual health. We need a sense of morality and virtue, not because the universe is clearly divided into good and evil, but precisely because it isn't.

Though it may not be apparent on the surface, our ongoing deliberations about whether, what, and how much to eat, along with the rules we create about food and our bodies, point to the need for this strong moral center. For without it, we are susceptible to *The Morality of Thinness,* whose laws about weight and eating are a superficial substitute for a true sense of integrity.

The Morality of Thinness is particularly tempting because it provides us with feelings of virtue, purity, and self-worth without our having to delve into the deeper issues of what it means to act ethically in our complicated world. Instead, we can simply deem ourselves "good" if we eat foods that are "good"—which, of course, means foods that help us get or stay thin. And we can always compensate for the "sin" of eating the "wrong" foods or eating "too much" by dieting, starving, overexercising, or purging. In the face of larger decisions that have no neat and tidy answers, this dogmatic, clear-cut, morality system not only makes us feel in control, it also makes us feel as though we are acting responsibly, even if our sphere of influence is reduced to the size of our bodies.

Unfortunately, when our sense of morality becomes intertwined with our devotion to thinness, the very commandments we obey in hopes of feeling virtuous become a source of self-judgment. We berate ourselves for not measuring up or for eating more than we "should." We feel guilty about skipping a day at the gym or for not being able to contain our appetites after going all day without eating. The result is that many of us live with a subtle, but ever-present, feeling of body shame. Indeed, this feeling is a cornerstone of The Religion of Thinness, which simply could not exist without it.

The real tragedy, however, is that our efforts to feel good about ourselves by focusing on the size or shape of our body divert our attention away from the most important ethical issues we face—both personally and as members of a global community. The Morality of Thinness reduces the scope of our decision-making to how we look and how many calories we consume. When body size becomes the grounds for proving our virtue, we lose sight of the pursuits that truly have meaning for us—pursuits that require us to care about something greater than the numbers on a scale.

If we want to stop condemning ourselves for failing to measure up to the implausible ideals of The Religion of Thinness and start living our lives from our *real* moral center, then we have to examine the spiritual needs that are concealed by our "right-and-wrong" approach to eating. In this chapter, I explore how The Morality of Thinness obscures these needs. I also show how it resurrects the long-standing religious legacy associating women, appetite, and sin, leaving us feeling either ashamed of our bodies or self-righteous when we compare ourselves to others. Learning to recognize and critique this legacy equips us to take the crucial step of developing an alternative perspective, one that helps us practice peace with our bodies by taking responsibility for our own well-being and serving the needs of the wider world.

Religion, Morality, and the Body

Morality has always been one of the primary concerns of traditional religions, which offer a variety of resources to encourage an upright life. Jewish ethics, for example, which are derived from the Torah, emphasize the responsibility of the entire community to abide by their covenant with Yahweh for the good of all Creation. Christians root their values in the teachings of Jesus, particularly his instruction to honor God and to love your neighbor as yourself. Several Eastern traditions follow the laws of karma, the belief that the present is shaped by past thoughts and actions, and that the future depends on current attitudes and behaviors. Both Hinduism and Buddhism incorporate the concept non-injury or nonviolence as a guide for moral conduct. "Truthful living" is the goal of life in the Sikh tradition, which advocates disciplined, personal meditation on the name and message of God. In Islam, the notion of *ihsan*, or "doing what is beautiful" reminds Muslims to act responsibly, which means not only that their behavior must be wholesome but also that their intentions must be good.

Although the moral vocabulary and emphases of religions differ, all suggest that we have a responsibility to act in an ethical manner and that human flourishing depends on doing so. This role cannot be understated. Spiritual and social leaders, such as Gandhi, Martin Luther King, Jr., Mother Theresa, and countless others used their faith as a foundation in their pursuit of peace and social justice. Many of us know of such people in our own communities—leaders of spiritual congregations, family members, co-workers, friends, teachers, social activists, and others—whose faith has inspired them to live a life of honesty, integrity, and service.

However, just as religions are sources of ethical values, they are also notorious teachers of *judgmentalism*: a black-and-white way of thinking that praises the "righteous" while damning the "sinners." Often this attitude finds its way into nonreligious contexts. Consider, for example, our culture's widespread condemnation of fat people as not only unhealthy but somehow depraved, as if the size of their bodies were an indication of some lack of inner virtue. Moral judgmentalism— whether or not it is explicitly religious—stems more from ignorance and fear than from knowledge or authentic faith. Criticizing others may provide the illusion of being superior, but in reality such a stance masks feelings of insecurity. It is when we are unsure of ourselves and out of touch with our moral center that we tend to solidify our sense of right and wrong, turning our opinions into laws and orthodoxies that require strict adherence.

These fear-based judgments are quite divisive and usually harmful. Those who abide by the code are "right," "good," "correct," "worthy." Those who do not are ostracized or considered "wrong" or "evil." Such thinking often plays out in clashes between people of different ethnicities, sexualities, or social classes, and even in the bullying behavior of school kids. It also permeates the history of religious wars and persecutions. The stories of heretics who were forced to convert or suffered burning at the stake illustrate how easily a moral code can be turned into an extreme way of thinking that, in its worst cases, leads to violence.

Whether or not we consider ourselves religious or accept the guidelines of traditional forms of faith, religions influence our decision-making because their general precepts permeate our society. Their influence is particularly strong when it comes to our bodies because the moral dictates of religion so often focus on regulating our physical appetites and urges. In Western culture, women's bodies and appetites have consistently been seen as sources of sin and temptation and thus in need of containment and redemption. This has had a tremendous impact on how women in this culture feel about and relate to their physicality.

The Legacy of Eve

One of the most influential stories of Western culture illustrates the supposed dangers of a woman's unruly appetite. In the bibilical story, humanity's fall from grace into sin is symbolically represented in the act of a woman eating. This tale has been told over and over again throughout the course of our history and it continues to influence attitudes towards women's roles and bodies today.[1]

The legacy of Eve not only equates the female appetite with temptation, but women themselves are cast into the role of temptress. After all, as the early Church Fathers were quick to point out, it was Eve who led Adam into sin, not the other way around. Many women today embrace, rather than contest, this ancient image of female-as-temptress by trying to create a "sexy" appearance. Even pre-adolescent girls know that dressing in a provocative way increases the likelihood that others will deem them "attractive" and thus worthy of attention.

Both girls and women adopt this role because it gives them a sense of self-worth that's missing in other areas of their lives. Feeling unimportant or unsatisfied in relationships, work, school, family, society, or religion drives many to seek a sense of self-esteem by creating an enticing appearance. The sad truth is that, despite the tremendous strides our culture has made with regard to gender equity, many of us still experience our bodies as the most readily accessible means for establishing our worth. Without knowing it, we have not only bought into the legacy of Eve, we have become trapped in it.

This legacy is duly complicated in that it not only dishonors women's bodies, it also offers the false promise of redemption through mastery of the flesh, self-sacrifice, and subordination to men. Women today "redeem" themselves by "purifying" their bodies: avoiding certain foods, suppressing their hungers, purging after bingeing, exercising to burn calories, and various other measures designed to create a certain appearance. In both the biblical story and in modern society's retelling of it, women are condemned to the flesh they must transform, and ultimately transcend, in order to be "good."

Although Christianity has had the most influence on Western attitudes toward women's bodies, it's not the only religion that perpetuates the links between women, physicality, and shame. The menstruation taboos of various traditions illustrate this view. In some branches of Judaism, for example, a menstruating woman can render a Jewish man unclean. In some contexts, Muslim women are forbidden to pray at that time of the month; and, in many tribal religions, women withdraw from their communities. Shinto women are prohibited from visiting sacred sites when menstruating. According to Pliny the Elder (23–79), an ancient Roman scholar, menstrual blood has such harmful power that it can cause iron to rust, wine to turn sour, beehives to die, dogs to go crazy, and crops to fail.[3]

Given the these time-worn associations, it's not surprising that women throughout history have turned to controlling their bodies as a means for cultivating purity and prestige in the eyes of others. One of the most striking examples of this can be found in the late Middle Ages in Christian Europe, where women engaged in behavior that some historians have referred to as "holy anorexia."[4]

Anorexia Mirabilis and the Power of Female Purity

Long before slenderness was the hallmark of beauty, some Christian women refused to eat or digest their food as a way to atone for their sins and the sins of others. In cases of prolonged abstinence, fasting was deemed miraculous. Later historical authors referred to this as *anorexia mirabilis:* the miraculous loss of appetite.[5]

One of the most famous holy women, Catherine of Siena (d. 1380), was said to subsist on the Eucharist (consecrated bread and wine representing the body and blood of Christ) alone. She reportedly stuck twigs down her throat to induce vomiting of any other food because she couldn't stand the feeling of anything else in her stomach. According to her biographer,

> The taking of food became to her not merely unnecessary but actually impossible, except to the accompaniment of great bodily suffering. If food was ever forced down her throat, intense pain followed, no digestion took place, and all that had been violently forced down was violently forced back again.[6]

Like other medieval holy women who fasted, Catherine believed that the pain of hunger connected her to the redemptive suffering of Christ. But refusing to eat did more than purify her body; it earned her the moral authority and public recognition rarely experienced by ordinary women of her time. In fact, the notoriety she gained by defying her appetite enabled her to intervene in the political and religious crises of her time, until she died of starvation.[7]

Christianity has a long history of asceticism, as discussed in the previous chapter. Certainly this was not restricted to women. Medieval Christian men also engaged in ascetic practices, but they were more likely to give up money, power, and prestige. Women seldom had the option of renouncing such things, as most were denied access to public debates and institutions. Being associated with physicality and sexuality, they were not encouraged to develop themselves intellectually. Instead, food and their bodies were the most readily available resources for exercising power and making the sacrifices that saintliness required.[8]

It's important to underscore the difference between medieval women's fasting and the eating problems of contemporary women. Medieval women were striving to be holy, not skinny. Today, women participate in The Religion of Thinness not out of devotion to God and service to others, but out of a desire for physical perfection, however much this desire masks a host of deeper spiritual needs.

At the same time, this obvious difference should not overshadow the links between them. Women of both eras have sought public approval through their bodies. And, although medieval women were not trying to be thin, their scrawny, shriveled bodies communicated to others an interior moral state of righteousness and virtue.[9] In the end, both the present-day quest for thinness and the medieval pursuit of holiness reflect a common struggle for purity and power in societies that view women's bodies as a source of immorality and shame.[10]

Internalizing the Legacy of Eve

Nowadays, women follow a set of regulations regarding their bodies that is no less strict than the ones followed by fasting women in the Middle Ages. This Morality of Thinness emphasizes how you look in relation to what, whether, and how much you eat, and its logic is seductively simple. Thin is good. Fat is evil. Consuming too much makes you immoral. Restricting intake makes you virtuous. There are good foods and bad foods, and the difference is measured in calories, fat grams, or carbs. Eating the wrong kind of food can make you impure. Eating the right food has the power to redeem.

Recognizing this state of affairs, eating disorder expert Carolyn Costin identifies our culture's "Thin Commandments":

1. If you aren't thin you aren't attractive.

2. Being thin is more important than being healthy.

3. You must buy clothes, cut your hair, take laxatives, starve yourself, do anything to make yourself look thinner.

4. Thou shall not eat without feeling guilty.

5. Thou shall not eat fattening food without punishing oneself afterwards.

6. Thou shall count calories and restrict intake accordingly.

7. What the scale says is the most important thing.

8. Losing weight is good; gaining weight is bad.

9. You can never be too thin.

10. Being thin and not eating are signs of true willpower and success.[11]

Even those of us living morally upstanding lives experience feelings of inadequacy when it comes to our bodies. A yo-yo dieter explained,

> I go to church every Sunday. I don't lie, cheat, or steal, and I give money to charity when I can afford it. Still, I can't help but feel ashamed of my body. I know I'm not that fat compared to some people. But even being a little overweight makes me feel guilty about eating…I find myself wanting to apologize a lot.

Many women live every day with a shaming voice inside their heads without ever fully realizing its impact. *"You're too fat," "You really need to lose weight," "You shouldn't have eaten this or that," "You'd be so much happier if you were thinner."* On and on this voice rattles and rants.

In her pioneering work with anorexics, psychiatrist Hilde Bruch asked her patients about this nagging inner voice. They described it as interfering with their hunger, as a kind of internal inquisition warning them not to eat and threatening them with images of fat. They characterized this judgmental voice in different ways, as "a dictator who dominates me," "a ghost who surrounds me," "the little man who objects when I eat." Interestingly, all of the women reported that the controlling voices in their heads were male.[12]

For young girls in particular, the values learned through The Morality of Thinness become foremost in their ethical thinking. In interviews with adolescent girls, for example, researchers Deborah Tolman and Elizabeth Debold asked a 7th grader to describe a recent conflict. The slender, blond girl reported difficulty in deciding, "whether I wanted the calories of two [pastries], or should I only have one." When pressed, the girl eventually revealed that her choice boiled down to, "whether or not I wanted the calories or to be good."[13]

These examples reveal the degree to which Eve's sinful appetite has become *our* sinful appetite. You may not sit around thinking, "I have the appetite of Eve; I better not eat this food, otherwise I will be sinning," but the ethical paradigm that you have unwittingly ingested—which leads you to moralize about food and criticize your body—reflects our culture's deep-seated association between women's bodies, appetites, and sin. These days, our disobedient cravings are punished neither by God nor any other external, "higher" being. Instead, we *chasten our rebellious appetites ourselves.* We feel guilty when we can't (or opt not) to repress our appetites, as if it were a sin to enjoy the mere pleasure of eating. We regulate, monitor, and mortify our bodies—not because we want to be holy, but because we want to be thin. Regulating our appetites becomes a way to absolve us of the shame of Eve: the disgrace of too much passion and the danger of too much hunger.

Depersonalizing the Shame: Critiquing the Corporate Underpinnings of The Morality of Thinness

Corporate entities across a broad spectrum of industries use The Morality of Thinness to promote their products. These companies use advertising strategies that deliberately tap into our desire not only to have a "good" body but to be a good person, and in many cases, they do so by employing the language and images of traditional religions.

This snack bar advertisement is a classic example: if we just eat the "right" thing—a Pure Protein bar—we can achieve an almost angelic state of purity.

In this ad there are two dominant images. The first is a slender, blond, blue-eyed woman, who appears to be in her late teens or early twenties, suited up in tight-fitting spandex and running shoes, jogging down a road. She is surrounded by puffy white clouds, suggesting that she is somehow in heaven. Her look is serene, her facial features almost angelic. She sports a golden halo. There isn't a drop of sweat on her face or a hair out of place. Even her running seems effortless. Indeed, she doesn't run, she floats through the air, apparently liberated from both the burden of her flesh and the gravity that keeps it earthbound. She has reversed the sin of Eve and is everything The Morality of Thinness encourages us to be: pure, disciplined, slender, good.

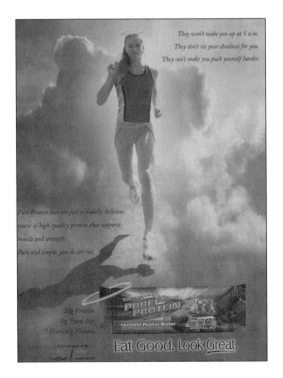

Pure Protein bar advertisement in *Women's Health* and *Fitness* magazines

The image of the Pure Protein bar just below her feet also wears a halo. The corporate slogan displayed in large type just under the holy bar reads: "Eat Good. Look Great." The nutritional details listed just to the left of the photo inform us that this bar contains "20g Protein – 0g Trans Fat – 7 Heavenly Flavors." (Never mind that this fat-free protein has been heavily processed). The message here is obvious: Pure Protein bars are just that—pure—and if you eat them, you will be too. More importantly, you will "Look Great" as a result of such virtuous eating. Indeed, your purity will be manifest in your lean and trim body—the visible index of your spic and span soul.

This message is both amplified and complicated in the text surrounding our fit little angel, which flows in almost poetic fashion. It reads:

> They won't wake you up at 5 A.M.
>
> They don't tie your shoelaces for you.
>
> They can't make you push yourself harder.
>
> Pure Protein bars are just a sinfully delicious source of high-quality protein that supports muscle and strength.
>
> Pure and simple, you do the rest.

While this might seem like a moment of "truth in advertising," the implicit assumption here is that we all *want* to wake up early and push ourselves harder, which is far from true. Or perhaps the more insidious assumption is that we *should* want to do this, which accomplishes what the ad was meant to do: fuel our feelings of inadequacy and drive us to eat Pure Protein bars, which of course, are "sinfully delicious."

Pure Protein's entire ad campaign (from their website to their television ads) revolves around this dance of temptation and redemption. Their TV ad features a woman in front of a bakery growing devilish horns as she contemplates having a pastry. The horns morph into a golden halo as she opts to eat a Pure Protein bar instead. Meanwhile, the voiceover says, "Pure Protein, a sinfully delicious treat for when temptation strikes."

Advertisements that rely on religious vocabulary seem to be particularly common in the marketing of diet or low-fat foods. For example, low-fat cream cheese is apparently a "heavenly" food, as the following ads insinuate:

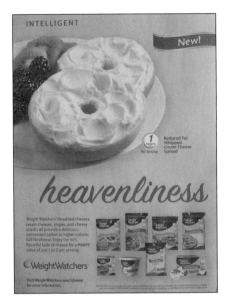

Weight Watchers advertisement

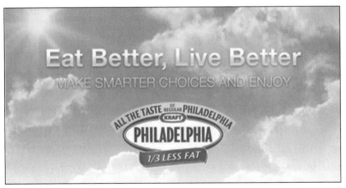

"Eat Better, Live Better" cream cheese advertisement

The Weight Watchers approach is unmissable with the headline of "heavenliness," but the Philadelphia cream cheese advertisement conveys a very similar message with its familiar celestial clouds. The bright white light in the upper left-hand corner of the image could be the sun; or perhaps it is the light of heaven itself. The headline of the ad informs us that we can live better if we eat better. This seems like a very good plan that Kraft is offering: we can enjoy ourselves more if we "make smarter choices" when it comes to food. Aside from the clouds and allusions to heaven, this ad doesn't *seem* to have much to do with The Morality of Thinness. It seems to promote healthy eating through conscious choices…until you look a little bit closer.

When you do, you may notice that the cream cheese advertised here has "1/3 less fat" than regular cream cheese. Granted, there's nothing inherently wrong with choosing reduced fat cream cheese. In fact, this may be the healthier choice for some of us. What's problematic is the way this advertisement quietly reinforces The Morality of Thinness by equating "eating better" with eating products that are reduced in fat (meaning products designed to help us get or stay thin), and this in turn is equated with "living better." To summarize this seductively simple formula:

eating better = eating low-fat = losing weight = living better.

Not only do these images connect "low fat" and goodness, but followers of The Religion of Thinness can deduce that regular food (i.e., whole or full-fat) is sinful. In fact, The Morality of Thinness tends to vilify whole or full-fat foods, while it glorifies foods that are highly processed to reduce caloric or fat content. This promotes a picture of "eating right" that is anything but healthy.

This ethical system reflects the kind of food orthodoxy that journalist Michael Pollan refers to as "nutritionism," according to which a food's nutritional value is based solely on invisible properties (e.g., vitamins, carbohydrates, fats, protein, etc.). Borne from an alliance between food marketers and nutritional science, this ideology convinces consumers of three harmful myths:

1. What matters most is not the food but the "nutrient."

2. We need expert help in deciding what to eat because nutrients are invisible and incomprehensible to everyone but scientists.

3. The purpose of eating is to promote a narrow concept of health.

Pollan challenges this conventional wisdom and the typical Western diet it has created (consisting largely of highly processed foods and refined grains which are grown with the help of chemicals in huge monocultures), arguing that this way of eating does little to foster our personal health or the wellbeing of our planet. In fact, as Pollan points out, much of what we're consuming these days is not really food, but "edible foodlike substances," the novel products of food science that come in packages often with health claims that frequently overstate their value.[14] Diet products are particularly well represented in this category. Most are aren't actually "foods" at all, but highly processed creations of human ingenuity engineered in laboratories with the aim of appealing to our taste buds and our desire to be "good" by losing weight. Many of the diet products we consume in an effort to be healthy would be unrecognizable to our ancestors. No wonder advertisers rely on the power of religious language to convince us of their benefits.

Understanding how the food, diet, and fitness industries resurrect the legacy of Eve to promote our culture's obsession with thinness can help us *depersonalize* the shame we feel about our bodies. Instead of assuming that our eating problems stem from our individual shortcomings and failures, we can begin to recognize the historical, religious, and commercial forces that contributed to their development. Practicing cultural criticism allows us to see that our seemingly-private preoccupations are part of a much larger history and social context.

This practice is especially important in a place where The Morality of Thinness has joined forces with a value system that many would not think to question: the Christian religion.

Critiquing Evangelical Christian Renditions of The Morality of Thinness

During the past decade or two, Christian-sponsored weight-loss programs have become wildly popular, offering an assortment of Bible-based books, workshops, and products that resurrect Eve's legacy in various ways.[15]

For example, Patricia Hill's *Slim for Him* likens the dangers of overeating to Eve's rebellious appetite. And in her "Weigh-Down Workshop," the largest devotional diet program in the world with 30,000 weekly meetings around the globe at its peak in popularity in the mid-1990s, Gwen Shamblin identifies feminine slimness as a sign of true Christian womanhood because it indicates that a woman has withstood the temptation to indulge her appetite and has submitted herself totally to God.[16] Shamblin actually preaches that eating too much is a form of rebellion against "Him." This, of course, implies that fat is an emblem of divine disapproval, a visible punishment for people who insist on putting food first.

Christian diet gurus proclaim varying messages. Some warn of God's wrath for those who indulge their cravings. Others emphasize divine compassion in spite of humans' sinful lack of restraint. Despite their divergent concepts of God, however, most leaders in the Christian weight-loss movement assume that "He" prefers us thinner, that being overweight is the direct result of overeating, and that fat is therefore a sign of perdition. Some say being fat is an indication of gluttony, one of the seven deadly sins. Others judge excess weight as evidence of idolatry, presuming large-bodied people worship food more than God.[17] Whatever their position, Christian evangelists for thinness share a common belief that the "sin" of overeating stems from individual weakness.

The titles of some Christian diet books—*Pray Your Weight Away; More of Jesus, Less of Me;* and *Help Lord! The Devil Wants Me Fat*—illuminate the extent to which The Religion of Thinness has infiltrated traditional religious beliefs and practices, and vice versa. The rules and mentality of devotional dieting are not easily distinguishable from the secular Morality of Thinness. As R. Marie Griffith notes in her analysis of Christian dieting, weight-loss evangelists like Shamblin have not been too concerned with the distinction between God's commands and society's norms.[18] Instead, they have increased the authority of our culture's dictates by turning them into divine decrees.

It's fairly clear that religious dieting movements like these only serve to reinforce the patterns of guilt and shame that are perpetuated by The Morality of Thinness. Focused exclusively on so-called individual fitness, the moral guidance they supply does nothing to increase the believer's sense of responsibility for anything beyond her stomach. But what may not be so clear on the surface is that the ideology underlying such programs gives them a frighteningly powerful marketing technique for those who create and sell them.

Consider what someone like Shamblin is doing. She taps into a Christian woman's desire for righteousness and redemption in the eyes of God by tying it to an idea that most women have been trained to believe since early childhood: that attaining the perfect figure will make them "good." She promises an answer for those who wish to please the Lord and get skinny all at the same time—her program. She further adds that failure to lose weight on her program indicates an individual's rebellion against God—rather than a problem with Weigh Down itself or the whole outrageous Morality of Thinness on which it is built. Insofar as she manages to sell this concept to women, she has consumers for life.

No matter how it's done, associating thinness with righteousness is reprehensible. When we assume a judgmental, moralistic division between those who are saved (thin) and those who are damned (fat), we aren't operating from anything resembling our true moral center. What we are actually doing is embracing a mindset that leads to violence.

How Fat People are Persecuted by The Morality of Thinness

Both males and females who are large-bodied are frequently subjected to emotional violence in the form of ostracism, scapegoating, and other forms of social derision that are a product of The Morality of Thinness. In her book *The Forbidden Body: Why Being Fat is Not a Sin,* Shelley Bovey quotes a number of women who describe the cruelty and discrimination they experience because of their size. One was told when applying for a job that the company had so many applicants that they didn't need to choose a fat one. Most of the 200 women Bovey surveyed said they were afraid to go to the doctor because of the insensitive or downright cruel lectures they received about their weight. One explained,

> Being fat is going to kill me, not because of the strain on my heart but because of the strain on my soul. I'm going to have some warning signs and avoid seeking health care until it is too late, because I am sick and tired of the canned speeches from doctors and nurses blaming my weight for everything.[19]

This woman's comment suggests that at least some of the health risks associated with being overweight may be better defined as social stigma than actual physical danger.

In this way, people of size endure a form of the bloodless violence perpetuated by The Morality of Thinness. They are frequently the targets of others' moral contempt. They are often judged and reproved by their peers, who see their "fat" as a manifestation of personal failure. A young woman who was struggling to accept her large body describes the pain this causes:

> All of my life, I have tried to accept the reality that my body is bigger than what's acceptable, and all of my life, I've had to listen to people tell me there's something wrong with me. I could fill a book with the names I've been called: "fat slob," "porky," "moo-moo," you name it. Even my own parents, who I know love me, can't help but feel ashamed of me. They sent me to a camp for fat kids when I was younger, and now that I'm older they're offering to pay for me to go for liposuction. It's hard to describe how much it hurts to have everyone look at you as though you're some kind of freak of nature.

Because fat people are viewed as personally responsible for the "sin" of their weight, they become convenient yardsticks for measuring and verifying the "piety" of their slender peers. Thus, we see another example of the dualistic, hierarchical thinking fostered by The Religion of Thinness: making you bad (because you're fat) makes me better (because I'm skinnier than you), and this gives me a (false) sense of self-worth.

In light of the subtle forms of violence fat people endure daily, it's not surprising that many of them resort to drastic measures, including lipo-suction or gastric bypass surgery, to make the "transgression" disappear. Weight-loss surgeries have become increasingly popular as new tech-niques are developed. Between 1993 and 2004, their numbers jumped 500 percent worldwide.[20] In 2007, well over 2.5 million women and girls under age 35 had some kind of cosmetic surgery to make them "more sexually attractive." In that same year, the total number of women who had their bodies surgically altered to "enhance their beauty" was closer to 5.5 million. The most popular surgery performed? Liposuction.[21]

Gastric bypass surgery is a particularly horrific procedure in which the lower part of the stomach is divided from the upper part by staples. The surgeon then connects a section of the small intestine to the pouch created by the staples—the upper, smaller part of the stomach. The purpose of the surgery is to shrink the size of your stomach so you will eat less. Though it is not generally recommended for cosmetic pur-poses, there can be little doubt that those who undergo it are fed up with being fat in a culture that demonizes obesity. In some cases of morbid obesity, the procedure may be perceived as life saving, despite the potential risks it involves, which include: anemia from vitamin B12 deficiency, internal bleeding, breakdown of the pouch which then needs repair, infections, malnourishment, and even death. A 2004 a study published in *The Journal of the American College of Surgeons* found that 2 percent of 3,328 patients who underwent the surgery died within the first 30 days after the gastric bypass was completed.[22]

In her book, *Hungry for More*, Robyn McGee writes about the loss of her beloved sister, Cathy, who died from complications related to gastric bypass surgery. According to McGee, it was Cathy's life-long dream to downsize her body from size 26 to size 9. Because she weighed 100 pounds over the "desired weight" for a woman her height, she qualified for the procedure. A few weeks before her unex-pected death she talked with excitement about a story she had read in *People* magazine about a celebrity's successful stomach-shrinking surgery. "With my operation," she proudly told her sister, "I'll be able to only eat cupfuls of food. I'll never be fat again!" Though it sounded risky, McGee didn't try to talk her sister out of the surgery primarily because she had seen how much Cathy had suffered throughout her life as a large-bodied black woman. Cathy never made it out of the hospital. She developed a post-surgical infection and died four days after the procedure. McGee concludes her account of this tragedy with the sad observation that her sister's "struggle with her weight was finally over."[23]

Most people who undergo gastric bypass surgery do so as a last resort. They feel there are no other options and are desperate by the time they make the decision. Who could blame them for their choice, given the social condemnation and derision they suffer daily as large-bodied people in a thin-obsessed culture?

And yet, as McGee points out, if we don't find a way to change what's in our hearts and minds, "no amount of surgery will make us feel whole."[24] Whatever health risks obese people experience as a result of their weight (and as we have learned, this relationship is dubious), we need to question whether surgery is really a road to a healthier body, mind, and spirit. What moral paradigm do we use to justify such a life-threatening procedure? What other alternatives are eclipsed by this "solution"? Is it possible that, as former U.S. Surgeon General Dr. M. Jocelyn Elders suggests, "a simple change of attitude—heightening self-love and self-acceptance—can prevent the need for life-risking surgeries and lead the way to healthier lifestyles"?[25]

Such thinking is contrary to The Morality of Thinness. For those who buy into this value-system, people with large bodies are infidels. And their heretical bodies *need* to be cut away. As abhorrent as this seems, such cruelty directed at people of size is an outward expression of the violence we do to ourselves when we judge our bodies based on The Morality of Thinness.

The Violence Within

Though people who have bought into The Morality of Thinness often judge others as a way to increase their sense of self-worth, their vitriol often reflects the shame they feel about their own bodies. A recovering bulimic woman illustrates this connection:

During those years of bingeing and purging, I really hated fat people because they reminded me of the part of myself that feels out-of-control. I also felt guilty for hating them, because I knew that if I hadn't found a way to get rid of everything I ate by vomiting and taking laxatives, I would look just like them.

Sometimes our image of God reinforces this domineering, moralizing attitude. Traditional views of the divine as an omnipotent being, a heavenly ruler, or the King of kings, define the ultimate power of the universe in terms of dominance and judgment, which are potentially violent postures. Such images reinforce the belief that we should control our bodies and that our unruly desires need to be punished—by any means necessary. Anthropologists who study religion suggest that sacred images provide models or patterns for relationships both *among* and *within* people.[26] If we envision God primarily as a judgmental ruler, we may be more likely to treat others and ourselves in a harsh, critical way: we condemn ourselves or others for being "too fat," accuse those who presumably "can't control their appetites" of being weak-willed or lazy, attempt to conquer our urge to eat by going on a diet, and chastise ourselves when we stumble.

Whether divinely influenced or not, the judgment that feeds this abusive behavior is the flipside of another violent moralizing tendency encouraged by The Morality of Thinness: the drive for perfection. It isn't simply that you need to be thinner than your peers to be righteous, you must have the *perfect* body, the one seen in the media. If you don't, you have failed. For some of us, this line between perfection and failure is *extremely* fine, as one woman's description of her eating problem suggests:

> I was on top of the world when I finally got down to a 107. Being 5'9", that weight seemed perfect for me. But whenever I ate too much and gained a few pounds, or even when I got my period and retained extra water, I felt totally miserable. I'd hurry my butt to the gym as fast as I could and I'd stay there until I was absolutely sure I'd burned everything off. I always liked it when people said I had a good body. But I doubt anyone had a clue about the pain I went through to maintain it.

When our sense of self-worth depends on being physically "perfect," the slope to failure is slippery and steep. A few pounds gained or lost become the difference between being a good or bad person. Our all-or-nothing approach to food and our bodies makes sense when the margin of error is so small: we either starve ourselves or eat with abandon, we either abhor our bodies or feel morally and physically superior, we either judge ourselves as total losers or fancy ourselves flawless. There is no middle ground.

Does classifying yourself as bad or good based on your size really reflect the value system you want to use in your life? Does passing judgment on your body and the bodies of others truly make you feel good inside? Or do such constant criticisms conceal deeper feelings of discontent, unworthiness, and fear? Maybe it's time to consider some of the needs that attract us to The Morality of Thinness.

Searching for a Moral Center in a Culture That's Out-of-Balance

Surely there is more to The Morality of Thinness than a desire to create a perfect body. Maybe our attempts to be "good" by repressing our appetites and reshaping our figures hide an even deeper desire to feel integrity in our lives, a sense that we are living our truest values. Perhaps our dichotomous, judgmental approach to weight and eating also masks an intense longing to move beyond the shame we feel. And, perhaps this shame is itself a signal that we've lost touch with our fundamental values and that we are morally out of balance. If this is true, then what The Morality of Thinness most reveals is our need to cultivate a strong moral center.

The truth is, we gravitate to this rigid value system because we have lost our ethical grounding—largely thanks to our culture's disordered priorities. Many of us tend to be self-absorbed. We are ambitious about our careers, determined to let nothing stand in the way of our success—not our relationships, not even our children, and certainly not the needs or concerns of people we've never met. Others lean in the opposite direction, being selfless to a fault by focusing exclusively on the needs of others while neglecting to nurture our own bodies and spirits.

Whatever your tendencies, following the codes of The Morality of Thinness is only likely to deepen your feeling of being out-of-balance because it *disconnects* you from your own moral center and from your responsibility to others.

This disconnection starts in our bodies. After years of obeying the dictates of our culture, most of us have long since lost the ability to listen to the wisdom of our flesh. And when we can't even manage to be accountable to what our bodies truly need, how can we expect to be fully present or responsible to the wider world?

Whether we are consciously running away from our ethical responsibilities by embracing The Morality of Thinness or unconsciously accepting the dictates of a society that encourages us to abdicate these responsibilities, the simple truth is this: the body itself is a source of great moral wisdom and the seat of our moral center. And it is by practicing peace with our bodies and retrieving this wisdom that we create harmony.

Retrieving the Wisdom of Our Bodies: Practicing Peace

You may not be aware of the role your body plays in moral decisions. However, our physical form impacts virtually all of our deliberations and the choices we make. This is not just because ethical decisions often involve bodily behavior (in terms of eating, sexuality, intoxicants, etc.). It's because our conscience develops and speaks through physical experiences. Consider the following:

Most of us know in our "gut" when something is wrong. We may get a headache when we're harboring resentment. Our heart may hurt when we're depressed or lonely. The kinks in our necks can be a sign that we're stressed or anxious. These are just some of the ways our conscience speaks to us through the wisdom of our bodies.

Listening to the cues our bodies send us is difficult when we've lived most of our lives ignoring, evaluating, correcting, and/or trying to control them. Because how we "should" look is based on societal norms, the energy we spend trying to improve our appearance dissociates us from our internal, physical experience. Moreover, years of observing the "Thin Commandments" (listed earlier in this chapter) have eroded our ability to sense when we're hungry or to know how much exercise we really need. It's hard to feel at home in a body that's always under surveillance. To reconnect with our body's wisdom, we must redirect our attention from how our body looks on the outside to how it feels from within.

This is where mindfulness exercises come into play. Practiced regularly, they strengthen the habit of living *in* your body and sensing your connection to the rest of the world. This not only increases your ability to recognize and heed the wisdom of your physical experience, it also deepens your sense of accountability to something larger than yourself.

The practice of listening to your intrinsic physical wisdom—paying attention to how your body feels on the *inside*—is a basic way to practice peace with your body. You can do this no matter what you are doing throughout the day. At work or at home, sitting down or being active, you can take a moment to notice how your body is feeling from within. Attending to, instead of ignoring or denying, these sensations guides us in making responsible choices about exercise and eating. As this interior awareness develops, we can begin to give ourselves the care we actually need, rather than acting based on what we think we *should* eat, how much we think we *should* exercise, or how we think we *should* look. Discerning the real needs of our bodies enables us to shift our focus from our physical *appearance* to our physical *experience*.

Attending to the real needs of our bodies is part of a larger spiritual process of becoming accountable to a reality that transcends our personal existence. It helps us develop the sensitivity and energy we need to be present to others. As body therapist Richard Strozzi Heckler states, "Experiencing the life of the body brings us into contact with the quality of compassion, something that is surely lacking in our troubled world."[27]

To live in our bodies is to be in touch with our capacity to feel. For it is in our bodies that we experience the suffering that softens our hearts and enables us to empathize with the pain of others. And it is through our flesh that we gain experiences that sharpen our critical awareness, enabling us to ask good questions and make responsible choices. And it is in our blood, our bones, our breath, our buttocks, that we come to know a passion that can energize our efforts to start living in a way that embodies our ultimate values.

Developing an Embodied Ethics of Eating

Reconnecting with the wisdom of our bodies empowers us to stop buying into the shame-inducing Morality of Thinness and look for more constructive, life-affirming ways to cultivate virtue in our lives. The more we pay attention to our bodies' internal sensations, intuitions, and feelings, the less reliant we will be on external rules and moralizing judgments to give us a sense of self-worth. As we grow beyond the mentality of The Religion of Thinness, we can embrace a more embodied ethic of eating: a nonviolent approach that emphasizes taking care of our bodies while also taking responsibility for our relationships within the wider circle of life.

Traditional religions have numerous examples of ethical codes that promote physical health and awareness while simultaneously reinforcing a sense of accountability and connection to sacred values. Most Hindus, as well as many Buddhists, observe a vegetarian diet as an expression of their intention not to harm themselves or others, including the earth. (Raising livestock for human consumption is one of the most significant contributors to a host of pressing environmental problems, including land degradation, climate change, air pollution, water shortage, and loss of biodiversity.[28]) Orthodox and many Conservative Jews follow kosher restrictions that originated in the Torah and are practiced for both sanitary and spiritual reasons. Traditional Buddhists avoid using intoxicants because of their propensity to increase the cravings that cause so much suffering in the world. Similar conventions can be found in the religious observances of both Mormons and Muslims, who refrain from alcohol, caffeine, and other such substances as a way to promote physical well-being and as an expression of their trust in God.

In different ways, these examples illustrate how we can embody our moral values through our everyday consumption patterns. As we reconnect with our bodies, we can use each choice as an opportunity to become mindful of what we "take in" and analyze whether or not it is a reflection of our true values. This goes not only for the foods we eat, but for the media we view, the people we associate with, and the thoughts and feelings we are exposed to (both internally and externally).

These choices determine the quality not only of our own lives but also of the world in which we live. We change the world by changing ourselves, one ethical decision at a time. We can begin small. I recommend starting with "A Day of Mindful Consumption."

A Day of Mindful Consumption: An Exercise in Developing Your Moral Center

In some traditional religions, one day of the week is set aside for spiritual contemplation. Perhaps the most obvious example is the Jewish and Christian tradition of the Sabbath. While many today do little more than attend synagogue or church, traditionally, the practice involves dedicating an entire day to rest, just as God is said to have rested (in the biblical narrative) on the seventh day after creating the universe. This observance offers believers an opportunity to spiritually center and replenish themselves, to reflect on their ultimate values and purpose in the grand scheme of things, and reconnect to their moral center. A Day of Mindful Consumption[29]—a day dedicated to practicing mindful awareness of what you take into your body, mind, and spirit—is a variation of this tradition.

Commit to One Day

Start by committing to this practice for one day. Think of it as a gift you are giving yourself. If you enjoy the exercise and find it useful, you may choose to do it more regularly. For now, just try it once as an experiment and see how it works for you.

On this day, your objective is to remain as conscious as you can of everything you let into your mind, heart, and body from the moment you awaken until you fall asleep at night. This includes your thoughts, feelings, and bodily sensations, the foods you eat and how they make you feel both mentally and physically, your interactions with others, the media you ingest, the beauty of silence, the experience of your breath, and the wonders of the natural world. The point of this exercise is not to judge yourself or your experiences; rather, it is to stay present to what your body is telling you about the options you have, the decisions you make, and the activities you enjoy.

To do this, you are probably going to have to *slow down* quite a bit from your usual pace of life. You need a day that's not dictated by an agenda or "to do" list, a day that doesn't require a lot of double-tasking. It's not that you're going to be inactive, it's that you do whatever you do consciously and fully. You may need to do this on a weekend or holiday.

If you have children, you might consider asking your partner, friends, or relatives to watch them. Or you could opt to spend your day of mindful consumption in the context of your ordinary family life. Depending on the age of your children, you might ask for their cooperation. This allows them to participate in your journey and gives them a wonderful example.

Start Your Day of Mindfulness

Once you've chosen your day to dedicate to mindfulness, figure out a way to remind yourself, at the moment of waking, of your commitment to spend the next 24 hours becoming more conscious about your choices. You could simply write the word "mindfulness" on a piece of paper and set it next to your clock. Or you might put an object on your bedside table (e.g., a picture, a rock, a bell, etc.) that reminds you to adopt a mindful stance as soon as you open your eyes.

Doing this will set the stage for being conscious of what you consume throughout your day. You can start by observing the breath coming in and out of your body. You may wish to count 10 slow, deep breaths as you lay in bed. As you do this, bring your attention to the way your body feels. Remember that this body is the temple in which you live and where you make decisions. Since you will be paying attention to whatever information your body gives you as you move through your day, you might begin this whole process by noticing where your body meets the sheets and blankets of your bed. Feel the soft pillow underneath your head.

As you arise, do so slowly. Notice the way your body moves from the prone position to an upright, seated posture. Feel the floor beneath your feet as you step on it. As much as possible, try to remain aware of your body's sensory experience—the feel of the carpet, the smell of the room, the light coming in from the window. See if you can notice some of these things as though for the very first time. As you do, become aware that you are ingesting these things all the time, but the quality of attention you bring to what you take in can significantly change the way it affects you.

Carry this mindful energy and the awareness of yourself as a consumer throughout your day. There are countless ways you might try to become more aware of the ideas and substances you absorb. Here are a just few suggestions that are specifically aimed at helping you remain more fully present in your body, and experience the wisdom it has to offer.

• Practice mindful eating

Each time you have a meal or snack, become mindful of the foods you eat. This is *very* different than counting calories or carbs. It's not about calculating what you take into your body; it's about actually *tasting* it and *feeling* it quench your thirst or ease your hunger.

Start by paying attention to your physical appetite, and examine what you *want* to eat. This could be anything from a pancake breakfast to a chicken dinner. Observe what your palate and stomach would most enjoy. Ask yourself: What kind of food would feel most satisfying? Try not to get caught up in a mental picture of what you'd like to eat (or what you think you "should" eat).

Once you decide what to eat, take time to prepare it with care. As you wash, cut, and cook the food, bring your attention to its smells and colors. Enjoy the sensuality of this experience. When you are done preparing your food, take a moment to notice what it looks like and how it is arranged on the plate. Express appreciation for it aloud or silently. What's important now is that eating is the only thing you are doing. (This means turning off the TV or putting down the book.) As you take the first bite, be aware of the flavors and textures of what you are eating. (Chewing slowly and completely is a helpful way to do this.) Take time to really *taste* what's in your mouth, and watch how your body responds.

After you have finished your meal, take time to notice whether or not the food you just ate makes you feel nourished physically, mentally, and spiritually. If you are prone to compulsive eating and find yourself craving more food, this is an excellent opportunity for you to sit with that feeling of craving, concentrating on your breathing, and remaining present to the urge until it gradually dissolves. Whether or not you try this tactic, try to let go of ideas about "good" and "bad" foods perpetuated by The Morality of Thinness and, instead, tap into the wisdom of your flesh. I don't encourage you to monitor your intake so much as to listen to the messages your body gives you. This can be difficult for those of us whose eating patterns have been oriented by a list of do's and don'ts. But with slow, attentive practice you can develop the capacity to hear and respond to your body's cues.

Eating foods that nourish your body and spirit is part of a healthy "way of life," which is what the word "diet" originally meant. As Buddhist teacher Thich Nhat Hanh suggests, the benefits of keeping our bodies healthy extend beyond our own personal interests:

> To keep your body healthy is to express gratitude to the whole cosmos, to all ancestors, and also not to betray future generations...If we are healthy, everyone can benefit from it—not only everyone in the society of men and women, but everyone in the society of animals, plants, and minerals.

"Health" in this context has nothing to do with a slender body. It has to do with living in harmony with your body's natural needs, the needs of others, and those of the earth. Practicing a "diet" of mindful eating is just one way to promote this harmony and the healing it brings.

• Mindfully consume media

Remember, what we ingest goes far beyond the foods we eat. Anything we take into our bodies, minds, or spirits, affects who we are. This, in turn, influences the world we live in. By mindlessly absorbing the media messages surrounding us, we inadvertently support the very industries through which The Religion of Thinness preaches its destructive messages.

I'm not recommending you throw your television out the window. I'm not even suggesting you completely opt out of consuming media during your day of mindfulness (though this may be a good option and one that will help you observe silence, as discussed below). I'm simply encouraging you to pay close attention to what you're taking in.

In fact, this is a perfect time to practice your skills in critical analysis. As you interact with media—whether it is the Internet, a magazine, or a movie—take the time to carefully and critically observe the messages you are encouraged to assimilate.

As you do this, you may find that a desire arises, very naturally from within, to expose yourself to other, more nurturing forms of culture instead. Follow that impulse. The more mindful we become, the more we will realize that many of the popular sources we have relied on to entertain us and help us relax—from MTV to *General Hospital*—leave us feeling unsatisfied. Spending a day practicing mindfulness can make us aware that what we really need is not more noise and visual stimulation, but a genuine way to rest and restore our spirits. A day of mindfulness is a good time to experiment with alternative ways of doing this. You might try turning off the lights and listening to soothing music, curling up on the couch with an inspiring book, or planting flowers in your back yard. Watch what happens within you—physically, psychologically, and spiritually—when you pursue alternative forms of recreation, replenishment, and pleasure. See whether they leave you feeling more grounded in your body and in the values you know to be sacred.

• Observe silence

One of the reasons we miss out on the beauty around us is because we are immersed in noise—from the sound of the alarm clock waking us up in the morning to the TV that dominates our evenings. We listen to the radio, talk on the phone, and endlessly babble with friends. Our society has lost touch with the power of silence. We don't know how to be still and listen. Are we afraid of what we might hear?

During your day of mindfulness you might choose to observe silence, either for the entire day or a portion of it. This could include refraining from talking, or leaving your radio and television turned off and listening instead to the silence that is always there but rarely heard. You may find it helpful to use the exercise from Chapter 1 and quietly sit, observing your thoughts and breath for one or more times during the day.

If you practice listening to the silence, you may hear a number of things that momentarily catch your attention: the hum of your refrigerator, the chirping of birds outside the window, the wind blowing through the trees, the clock ticking on the wall. These sounds of silence can be pathways back to the present, back into this moment just as it is.

• Gently and persistently bring yourself back to the present

If you have tried any of the mindfulness exercises in this book, you are well aware that it is difficult to remain fully present even for a few moments. How can you expect to be mindful for a whole day?

Remember, mindfulness is a practice—a process—not an end product or destination. You won't remain mindful every minute of the entire day. It is natural to get caught up in your thoughts and feelings, whether they are about food, your body, or anything else. That's completely normal and I urge you not to judge yourself. The point is not to remain perfectly mindful. The point is to use this day as a chance to practice a skill that can help you strengthen your sense of accountability to yourself and others. In so doing, you may learn to enjoy your life in a whole new way. But beating yourself up for "not being mindful enough" will only further alienate you from the moral center you need to develop.

When you catch yourself getting hooked by thoughts about your "fat" thighs or what you "should" eat for dinner, gently and persistently bring your attention back to the present. There's no need to fight your thoughts or feelings. The goal is not to exorcise them, but to accept them for what they are—just thoughts and feelings. You don't have to judge yourself for having them. You don't have to act on them either. Part of the beauty of this day is that you have all the time you need to *notice* the urges that feel desperate or the emotions that feel destructive, and to *pause* before letting them envelope you. This is not about suppressing anything. It's about interrupting the momentum of your habitual responses, whatever form they take. It is an act of kindness towards yourself and the world of which you are a part.[30]

This is the compassion that is necessary for healing. I encourage you to forgive yourself for the ways you have acted that are not aligned with your truest values. Shaming yourself is never helpful, much less healing. Instead, treat yourself with the same sensitivity and care you would give a small child who is crying in your arms. You've been hurt by the world and have developed a hurtful relationship with your body in response to this pain. Now you have a chance to start the process of healing. This is a moral path of compassion and love, not guilt and punishment.

• Reflect on your thoughts and feelings

Toward the end of the day, take some time to reflect on what you have experienced and write down your impressions. How do your patterns of consumption affect your health? How do they affect the health of our planet? How might you become more mindful of and responsible for the choices you make on a daily basis? How might you orient your everyday choices in ways that contribute to the common good?

Questions like these help us remember that our mundane choices affect our own well-being and reverberate around the planet. Our obsession with calories and thinness may blind us to the consequences of our actions and perceptions, which have the potential to injure not just ourselves, but others. A Day of Mindful Consumption helps us break out of the prison of self-absorption that this preoccupation has constructed. At the same time it nurtures us in ways that may be missing from our stressful, hurried, daily lives. Devoting a day to practicing mindful consumption allows us to develop an alternative ethic, one that helps us stay grounded in our bodies and makes us aware of the connections between the choices we make, our personal well-being, and the welfare of others and, ultimately, our planet.

Moral Lessons from the Earth

As we look for resources to help us strengthen and live from our moral center, we might turn our attention to the natural world. Like our own bodies, the earth is an abiding font of wisdom. Trees, for instance, can be great teachers. Just imagine the grace of a tall palm tree, leaves flowing freely like long hair in the wind. Then consider the beauty of a sequoia, with its thick trunk, furry bark, and drooping branches. Each is beautiful in its own way. How silly it would be to wish that one looked more like the other.

In one of the scenes from her play, *The Good Body,* Eve Ensler depicts a conversation she had with a 74-year-old African Masai woman named Leah, who is trying to understand America. She asks:

> Leah: What kind of place is it? In Africa, we are desperate for food, we have so little; in America, where you have all the food, you either eat too much or not at all. Your bodies are just pictures to you. Here we live in our bodies, they serve us, they do our work.

When Eve explains how impossible it is for her to appreciate her own body, especially her stomach, Leah is genuinely puzzled: "What's wrong with it?" she asks.

> Eve: It's round. It used to be flat.

> Leah: It's your stomach. It's meant to be obvious. It's meant to be seen. Eve, look at that tree. Do you see that tree? Now look at that tree. *(Points to another tree)* Do you like that tree? Do you hate that tree 'cause it doesn't look like that tree? Do you say that tree isn't pretty 'cause it doesn't look like that tree? You're a tree. I'm a tree. You've got to love your body, Eve. You've got to love your tree. Love your tree.[31]

Perhaps one of the reasons we agonize so much over our tummies, or whatever body parts make us suffer, is that we are so alienated from nature. We need to return to this wellspring of wisdom, to let the lessons of the earth instruct us. In nature, there is nothing to compare ourselves to, no human-made standard by which to measure ourselves. The trees, the tides, the sky, and all the other life forms that surround and support us have a remarkable tendency to accept things as they are and as they change. Does the sky regret the sunset because its beauty ends?

Like the wisdom of our bodies, the insights of the natural world are always available to us. Even if you live in the city, there is always the sky to put things in perspective, and the ground you walk on to help you feel supported. Wherever you live, I recommend spending as much time as possible in the beauty of nature. Go for a slow, gentle hike in the woods, leisurely walk along the beach, or simply spend time sitting on a bench in the park. As you do, be mindful of your surroundings. Study the trees and their branches. Listen to the sound of the wind in their leaves, or the tide breathing in-out-in-out. Feel the grass or sand beneath your feet. Appreciate the warmth of the sun or the cool of the breeze. Look up at the sky. See the clouds. See the blue. Let the beauty of these things inspire you to find your way back to your heart's deepest truths.

A sun-sparkling lake or trickling stream can put us in touch with that peaceful place somewhere deep inside us, that part of us that is content to be who we are. A thunderstorm can remind us of our inner wildness that refuses to be manipulated and tamed into being a "proper" lady. The grandeur of mountains can help us put things in perspective, reminding us how small our problems really are in the greater scheme of things. Most of us need the mirror of nature to help us see ourselves and the world more clearly: to find tranquility in the midst of life's chaos, beauty amid its diversity and "imperfections," and truth within its interconnections.

Strengthening our relationship to the earth is a fundamental way to stay grounded in our bodies while cultivating a sense of environmental responsibility. The natural world is the body on which our bodies depend, and our relationship to the earth reflects our relationship to our own physical form. Treating our endangered planet with respect and kindness through acts as simple as recycling or using less water teaches us to nurture our own well-being and to be sensitive to the needs of others. Encounters with nature remind us that the world is much greater than The Religion of Thinness would have us imagine, and that we have a responsibility to care for all forms of life.

Recognizing Our Interconnection within the Larger Web of Life

This moral task may seem impossibly large. How can we even hope to change the decay of our planet—or anything else for that matter—when we're preoccupied with calories and thinness? How can we work to heal the world when we can't seem to heal ourselves?

Keep in mind that caring for the earth and transforming our relationship to food and our bodies are intertwining, not opposing, tracks. For perhaps more than any other daily activity, what we eat connects us to the rest of the world. It is impossible to drink a cup of coffee without indirectly touching the lives of countless strangers, from the people across the globe who grow and harvest the beans to those responsible for delivering our favorite brand to the grocery store. Thich Nhat Hanh describes the fundamental interdependence of life like this:

> A piece of bread contains a cloud. Without a cloud, the wheat cannot grow. So when you eat the piece of bread, you eat the cloud, you eat the sunshine, you eat the minerals, time, space, everything.[32]

Living responsibly in light of our interconnection with the earth and with others begins with the small, ordinary choices we make about food and our bodies. To consider the consequences of these decisions both on and beyond your personal sphere, you can expand the practice of mindful eating discussed earlier to include reflection on the origin of your food. Where did the banana you eat grow? Who harvested it? Who drove the trucks to market? Is the chicken you will have for dinner from a factory or a free-range farm? Are the vegetables you eat organic or are they conventionally grown with pesticides and other chemicals that compromise your health and pollute the earth? As you reflect on the differences between these options, watch what thoughts and feelings come up. Being mindful of where your food comes from is a way of deepening your sense of connection to—and responsibility within—a global community.

There are countless opportunities for promoting our own health while contributing to the sustainability of the planet. Every time we go grocery shopping or eat in a restaurant, we can select foods that are fresh or unprocessed and that are grown and harvested in ways that don't damage the earth's ecosystems. Choosing foods closer to their original state, including whole grain, organic, and locally grown foods, tends to be better for both our health and the environment. Foods that are locally grown are not only fresher, but require less of the earth's resources to get to our table. It seems incongruous that produce in the average grocery store in the U.S. travels nearly 1,500 miles between the farm where it was grown and your refrigerator.[33] As conservationist Jane Goodall reminds us, "Every food purchase is a vote…each meal, each bite of food, has a rich history as to how and where it grew or was raised, and how it was harvested."[34] These purchases, these day-to-day "votes," involve moral decisions that will determine the health of our individual bodies and the future of our natural environment.

When our food choices are dictated by the imperative to create a "good body," we may stress all day about calories and carbohydrates without considering where our food comes from, what chemicals have been added to it, how much it has been processed, or whether it has been genetically modified to withstand higher levels of pesticides, or whether the people who grew and harvested it were justly compensated. Developing our moral center means expanding our ethical universe not only beyond The Religion of Thinness but also beyond our personal self-interests, so that we clearly see the process of our own recovery as inextricably connected with healing the planet.

This shift implies a new understanding of sin, one that redirects our attention away from the narrow sphere of personal indiscretions to the larger cultural milieu whose social injustices and materialistic values jeopardize every person's well-being. In this broader perspective, it's not our appetites that are sinful, but the cultural norms, industries, and institutions that perpetuate the legacy of Eve by encouraging us to feel ashamed of our bodies.

Sin in this view is also manifest in the injustices that permeate the global food supply. There currently exists enough food to feed every child, woman, and man a diet of 2,500 calories a day. Yet nearly half the world's population suffers from malnutrition. According to the United Nations, 18,000 children die each day from hunger.[35] As theologian L. Shannon Jung observes, the global food system fails to respond to such preventable suffering because it prioritizes corporate growth, consumer spending, and profitability over human well-being. Its goal is not keeping our bodies healthy, but finding ways to entice us to consume more than we really need. It enables those of us who live in well-developed countries to eat food that is relatively convenient and cheap. But it does so by overtaxing the earth's ecosystem, using up its renewable resources faster than they can be replenished, and pouring chemicals into the soil to increase productivity. The wealthiest nations are the most responsible for the ecological havoc this system is creating. The richest 15 percent of the earth's population uses 75 percent of its energy, a good portion of which is for growing, transporting, and fertilizing crops.[36] *We* are responsible for this.

Widening the Scope of Our Awareness and Compassion

The key to living a life from our moral center is shifting our paradigm from judgment to responsibility. This requires us to see our "personal" thoughts and behavior around weight and eating in relation to something larger than our individual bodies. As we widen the scope of issues we deliberate about when making choices about what, whether, and how much to eat, there are a number of ways we can become more accountable to the welfare of others. We may give our time, energy, and money to causes that aim to eradicate world hunger. For example, as part of her healing, a woman who had spent years battling her weight made a commitment to donate the same amount of money she spent on "fixing" her body to organizations that serve undernourished children. Every time she purchased an item to improve her appearance—from mascara, to hair coloring, to clothing designed to make her look thinner—she contributed the same amount of money to organizations such as OXFAM or UNICEF (*www.oxfam.org* and *www.unicef.org*).

Some of us may feel called to take a more active role in our most passionate causes. For example, one woman who ate compulsively in front of the TV at night began volunteering at a women's shelter several evenings during the week instead. The more involved she became in the lives of the women and children there, the less she found herself obsessing about food and the size of her body. She explained:

> My work at the shelter hasn't 'cured' me of my eating problem, but it has changed the way I look at myself and the world. Basically, it's made me a lot more aware of other people's needs and struggles. I guess you could say it's also given me a deeper satisfaction than I've ever experienced from eating.

Becoming morally responsible by serving others is not just a matter of doing "charity." Rather, it is a way of meeting our spiritual needs and seeing how our own well-being is inextricably linked to the welfare of others. Considering the influence that your eating and exercise habits have on young girls—your daughters, granddaughters, sisters, nieces, or students—may make you think twice about skipping meals or spending hours at the gym in order to make yourself feel virtuous.

There are numerous ways to extend your energies and talents in the service of others as part of your recovery process. You may start or join organizations that aim to promote healthy body image by critiquing our culture's devotion to thinness. In the mid-90s, for example, a group of former anorexic and bulimic girls and women, along with their therapists and mothers, formed an activist coalition called Boycott Anorexic Marketing (BAM). This grassroots group successfully pressured the Coca-Cola company to withdraw a Diet Sprite ad that featured a gangly young woman called "Skeleton." Therapist Mary Baures, who started BAM, explained that its aim was not simply getting anorexic advertising removed, but also giving women and girls who felt powerless a way of getting back their voices.[37]

About Face is a similar organization that is alive and thriving today (*www.about-face.org*). The organization was born in 1995 when Kathy Bruin plastered hundreds of posters critiquing anorexic marketing in the San Francisco area. Its current goals include: empowering people of all shapes, colors, cultures, and ages to feel confident about their bodies, encouraging healthy skepticism about media images and the messages of popular culture, educating the public on subjects of sexism, looksism, and weight obsession, creating alternative images through posters and art installations, and using playful and original ideas to generate cultural critique and change.[38]

Parents have a fundamental role to play in helping their children make responsible decisions with regards to food. In addition to setting a good example by treating their own bodies with care and respect, parents can advocate on behalf of their kids for a culture that promotes healthy eating patterns. One band of concerned moms and dads in the small city of Moorhead, Minnesota, for example, pooled their intelligence, energies, and time to lobby the local school district to provide more nutritious school lunches for their children. Members of this grassroots group, called Concerned Parents for School Nutrition, had noticed that a number of items on the school lunch menus shared similarities with fast food. The group encouraged their school district to go beyond meeting the minimal USDA guidelines for school nutrition and to include in the school lunches foods that are organic, non-irradiated, and locally grown or produced. While their goals are not directly intended to dismantle The Religion of Thinness, they are connected to this cause because they aim to promote life-long healthy eating habits and ecological sustainability.

Beyond the Good Body

Participating in such grassroots efforts supports our own well-being and the health of others. By becoming involved in moral causes beyond that of creating a "good body," we transform the shame that prevents us from fully living into energy for our journey of healing.

What does it mean to be "good?" Does it really depend on repressing our appetites and sacrificing our pleasures? Is that what it takes to have a "good body"? Is a "good body" essential for being a "good" person? In the concluding monologue of *The Good Body*, Ensler ponders these questions, and suggests:

> Maybe being Good isn't about getting rid of anything.
>
> Maybe good has to do with living in the mess
>
> in the frailty
>
> in the failures
>
> in the flaws.
>
> Maybe what I tried to get rid of is the
>
> goodest part of me.
>
> Think Passion.
>
> Think Fat.
>
> Think Age.
>
> Think Round.
>
> Maybe good is about developing the capacity
>
> to live fully inside everything. . .[39]

The Morality of Thinness hooks us by appealing to our desire to feel virtuous and worthy, and we cling to its rules and standards because we have lost touch with our innermost selves. We practice reconnecting with those values through our daily decisions. Each time we choose to eat in ways that respect our bodies rather than listen to the shaming voices outside and within us, we strengthen our connection to what we deem sacred. Step by step, our disobedience to The Morality of

Thinness becomes a virtue, rather than a sin, as we make choices that challenge a moral system that makes us feel homeless inside our own bodies. Such choices reverse the legacy of Eve, paving the way for both ourselves and others to heal.

6

FROM CONFORMITY TO SELF-ACCEPTANCE

"The Community of Thinness" and Our Need for Unconditional Love

"One-and-two-and-three-and-four, kick and step and touch the floor." Diane tried to keep up with the aerobics instructor on the platform. She imagined how good it would feel to be so lean, how gracefully her body would jump and move, how much easier her life would feel. Looking around, it seemed that everyone in the class was thinner than she was. How could this be?

Her mind wandered to her husband, whose moodiness had reached a crescendo of late, making it difficult to be around him, much less feel connected in any kind of intimate or meaningful way. This, the seemingly-constant pressure at work, and the daily demands of their children had become too much. She constantly found herself feeling frustrated, resentful, and alone.

Diane's thoughts were interrupted. This was the part of the combination she loved most: the dance-like movement that sent the entire class of women whirling in unison to the left, then to the right. As the music pulsed, she took a deep breath and felt momentarily transported. For that instant, she stopped comparing herself to the women around her and felt connected to them as they all moved together as one.

But the moment was short-lived.

If you have spent time practicing The Religion of Thinness, chances are you are quite skilled in the art of comparing your body (or body parts) to those of other women.

Ironically, this competition is also a means for bonding. We connect in conversations about our "need" to trim down, our success or frustration in this endeavor, our guilt when we eat some high-calorie food, or our observation that someone "looks so good" since she's lost weight. These discussions are a source of both pain and pleasure, both bondage and communion, depending on how well we are measuring up.

In the end, however, our comparisons and conversations mask a deeper need for relationships that can support and sustain us throughout our lives.

Human beings are social creatures. We need more than food and shelter to truly thrive. Each of us needs to be part of a community—a group of people with whom we share a history or common values, interests, and goals. We need to experience ourselves as belonging to something bigger than ourselves, something we can depend on when our lives feel shaky, that channels our energies beyond our small selves, that encourages our spiritual strivings, and that enables us to experience love in spite of our problems and imperfections. This is what community offers, and when it functions well, it is a remarkable gift.

Unfortunately, in our efforts to feel a sense of belonging, many of us have become part of a "community" that doesn't direct our attention to anything larger than the size of our bodies. The support it offers is highly conditional, and the values it affirms do not resonate with our deepest wisdom. Its common cause is nothing more than a "better body."

Though it has no official title, no formal mission statement, no central headquarters, and no clearly defined organizational boundaries, The Community of Thinness is vaguely comprised of a "group of believers" who, despite their cultural, political, educational, economic, and religious differences, seek and find support from each other in their common goal of a slender figure. This sense of community is fostered through a variety of mechanisms, including commercial weight loss programs, a shared language, initiation experiences that create the reassuring feeling that "we're in this together," and ritualized confessions that make us feel accepted despite our food and body "failures."

Many of us believe that people will love us more if we are thin. We imagine that we'd be more popular and have more friends if our bodies more closely resembled the cultural stereotype of beauty. Or we may turn to weight-loss as a strategy for finding love, believing our success in romance depends on it.

On the other hand, there are those of us who engage in obsessive eating or exercise behaviors either to avoid or as a substitute for the relationships we really need. It is not uncommon for women to turn down social engagements because they think they're "too fat" to be seen in public, or because they feel compelled to stay home and binge. "Unlike people and social situations," a woman who struggled with compulsive eating explained, "food is a reliable source of comfort."

Most of us could use a little more love, nurturing, and acceptance in our lives. But when we search for these things in relationships that revolve around food and thinness, we are likely to end up feeling even more isolated and lonely. Bonding over food and weight-loss may temporarily relieve such feelings, but The Community of Thinness is a double-edged sword. It encourages us to relish the praise we receive when we lose weight, but it also causes us to fixate on the disapproval we get when we gain. Even more to the point, when our friendships revolve around the common quest to be thin and we spend a lot of energy comparing ourselves to the very women with whom we wish to connect, it becomes virtually impossible to develop meaningful relationships.

Our shame festers in isolation, and this is a heavy cross to bear. It isn't until we break our silence and begin conversing with others—especially those who are capable of loving us unconditionally and who are conscious of cultural influences—that our experience begins to change. By doing this we take another step toward freeing ourselves from The Religion of Thinness and start learning how to feel good about our bodies.

This chapter brings our desire for supportive relationships into focus by highlighting why we need to feel connected and the various ways we try to fill this need through The Religion of Thinness. It explores how The Community of Thinness functions to create a sense of belonging through the use of traditionally religious rituals like our "confessions" about eating. It shows how our attempts to conform our bodies to a widespread but narrow ideal conceal a desperate attempt to feel accepted and affirmed in a society where traditional ties have been weakened or broken. And it examines how the competitive nature of The Religion of Thinness robs us of the connections we need to sustain us, making us feel jealous instead of joined. Finally, it explores some options for developing alternative relationships that offer the genuine love and support we need to leave The Community of Thinness behind, heal the wounds it has inflicted, and learn to accept and love ourselves as we are.

Our Need for Supportive Relationships: Religion as a Communal Affair

A variety of religious traditions have provided crucial resources for addressing the human need for community, and they continue to do so today. Synagogues, mosques, temples, monasteries, ashrams, and churches are all gathering places where people have historically sought to experience a sense of belonging. This feeling is particularly important in times of celebration or loss.

Christians usually celebrate the birth of a child by gathering for the infant's baptism, a ritual of initiation into the community. Jews celebrate a child's coming of age with a Bar Mitzvah (for boys) or a Bat Mitzvah (for girls), thereby becoming privileged to participate in all areas of Jewish life. In some cultures, Buddhists congregate at the gravesite of a loved one on the anniversary of her or his death to commemorate and connect with the life of their ancestor. Muslims from around the world make a pilgrimage to Mecca every year to share their common devotion to God. For Muslims, the *ummah*, which is the community of believers, is the primary source of identification, transcending all other loyalties and bonds.

The importance of identifying with a community is particularly strong in Native American traditions, where one's own personal identity means little apart from one's tribal connection. In his autobiography, for example, Black Elk (1863–1950), a shaman of the Oglala Sioux, describes how he was given the same name as his father, as well as his grandfather and great grandfather.[1] Individual identity is not an important part of this culture where one's own well-being cannot exist apart from the health of the community. Among First Nation peoples, "community" extends to the natural world to include animals, trees, rocks, rivers, and insects, as well as ancestors and other spirits. To separate ourselves from the web of life (both human and otherwise) that sustains us is, in this worldview, inherently self-destructive.

While religions provide resources for meeting our need for belonging, communities do not have to be religious to offer support and a sense of connection. A variety of social groups such as athletic teams, political parties, professional organizations, and book clubs address our need to be part of something that transcends our individual lives. The Community of Thinness does not.

The Community of Thinness and the Illusion of Connection it Fosters

We are drawn to The Community of Thinness for the same reasons that some people belong to a religious community: to feel connected both to a larger purpose and to others who share our beliefs. Each of the mechanisms used to create The Community of Thinness (e.g., initiation rites, shared language, confessions, etc.) parallels methods used in traditional religious communities to create this sense of belonging. We will analyze these parallels throughout this chapter, but let's begin by considering one of the most obvious examples: the commercial weight-loss programs that promise their members not only the tools they need to reshape their bodies, but also the support required to sustain their spirits.

Commercial Weight Loss "Communities"

A typical Weight Watchers meeting resembles the services of some churches. The leader, who functions like a minister, shares her "conversion" story, describing the misery of her former life as an overweight person and offering strategies for successful weight loss and maintenance. She may give advice from the company's philosophy and highlight the value of its various products. When she finishes telling her story, she invites others to testify about what works for them. Those who do reinforce their feeling of belonging.

"There is a sense of community at these meetings," a member explained. "We're all working on a common problem, and we support each other in our victories and failures. I like knowing that I'm not the only one with a problem, and that there are people I can go to when I need help, people who accept me even when I screw up."

On the surface, the kind of community Weight Watchers fosters through its quasi-religious meetings may seem quite positive. After all, isn't it a good thing that members "support each other in their victories and failures" and feel as though "there are people they can go to when help is needed." Isn't this what communities *should* offer? To answer these questions we must use our critical eye and ask ourselves who stands to gain when people join the Weight Watchers community. When we do, it's easy to see that the corporation's motives are anything but altruistic. It's a *business*—the largest weight loss corporation in the world. To think they have altruistic motives would be naïve.

One of the key methods for achieving success through their program is their meetings, which are featured on their website. Click through to the "Community" page, and the first thing you see is this banner:

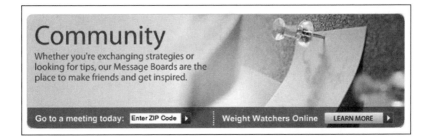

Detail from Weight Watchers website

As you can see, the text reads, "Whether you're exchanging strategies or looking for tips, our Message Boards are the place to make friends and get inspired." Just below this you are invited to locate a Weight Watchers meeting near you. Once you do so, you are taken to a page that lists groups in your area. I live in the upper Midwest in a relatively rural part of the country, but when I enter my zip code, 10 meetings are instantly located. If you live in an urban area, you can find dozens, as many as 100 meetings per zip code, which is the stated limit.

On the page where meetings in your area are identified, the "10 things you should know about meetings" are also listed.

1.   Each weigh-in is confidential.

2.   Meetings work for both men and women.

3.   There are no required foods…eat what you like.

4.   Meetings are dynamic, diverse and fun.

5.   Leaders have lost weight with Weight Watchers.

6.   You don't have to talk if you don't want to.

7.   It's easy to find a meeting near you.

8.   There are lots of meeting times to choose from.

9.   Weight Watchers eTools is available.

10. There are many flexible payment options to choose from.

Despite the obvious marketing ploys inherent in the language in this list, the appeal is intended to get you to sign up, because joining the program has the benefit of linking you to a community of others who also want to lose weight. And, connecting with these potential new "friends" increases your chances of success.

The weigh-in at the start of meetings is an important means for creating this solidarity. It is a ritual everyone goes through and does not appear to be optional. Even though it's "confidential," a weigh-in is likely to bring up feelings of shame for women who have struggled with overeating. Even when the number on the scale is "good news" (i.e., pounds have been lost), shame is still part of the equation—only in this case, it is temporarily pacified by the feeling that you are making progress. Whether the weigh-in ritual triggers or tempers your shame, it is ultimately designed to make you want to buy Weight Watchers products, which the leader in the meeting will be happy to sell you. Most of these leaders aren't volunteers from the community. They are paid a flat fee plus commissions for running meetings and selling products.

The meetings themselves aren't free either. The "many flexible payment options available" include paying by the week or purchasing the "Monthly Meeting Pass." This pass entitles you to as many meetings as you want to attend for a set monthly fee, which you can pay with your credit card on a renewing basis—a ploy that allows them to continue taking your money even if you don't attend meetings and are too shamed to actually quit and stop the credit card charges.

Not only are there many meetings near you at a variety of times, Weight Watchers also brings meetings to your workplace with their "Weight Watchers at Work" program. This is another effective marketing tool for this immense corporation. Their advertising encourages you to start a "Weight Management Group" at your office, which not only gives you greater convenience, but also "the power of group support." The marketing of this program—which is aimed across ethnic, racial, and gender lines—reinforces the message that taking your weight loss goals to work increases your chances of success, satisfaction, and inclusion. Also, since most people spend "the bulk of their day on the job," why not convert the daily drudgery of life at the office into an opportunity to shed pounds?

Hasn't The Religion of Thinness already absorbed enough of your waking hours?

The reality is that many of us are stuck in jobs that feel meaningless or unfulfilling. The endless hours we put in at the office not only deplete our energy but also leave us feeling disconnected—both from other people and from our larger values and aspirations. The Weight Watchers at Work program appeals to this disconnection, but, ultimately, it cannot resolve it. Like other examples of The Community of Thinness, it creates the feeling of inclusion by keeping you fixated on a common goal that has nothing to do with your life's true purpose.

You don't have to feel bad about yourself if you've tried (or are trying) the Weight Watchers program. As I've pointed out, on the surface it seems quite sensible. It claims that it won't tell you what you should eat, and it offers the support you know you need. In fact, there's a healthy instinct behind the decision to join such a program. A person who does may realize that her struggle with food is too big to handle by herself; she may recognize her need for fellowship with others who are similarly seeking to resolve this struggle. The trouble is that programs like Weight Watchers tend to exacerbate—rather than alleviate—our preoccupation because they fail to challenge the paradigm that makes weight the problem and thinness the solution.

Of course, Weight Watchers isn't the only diet company that uses meetings as a marketing tool. Other commercial weight loss programs and virtually every new diet that comes on the market have established so-called communities people can join. These fellowships are often one of the chief components advertised by these programs, and their promises are universally the same: this community will help you stick to the plan and lose weight. Such promises are also universally deceptive. They entice you with the hope of meaningful friendships and supportive connections, but they also feed into the larger economic paradigm of The Religion of Thinness. Remember, healthy communities support and inspire their members rather than routinely shame them by systematically stirring the very issues that cause the most pain. A healthy community does not prioritize commercial gain over the well-being of the members it serves.

Initiation into The Community of Thinness

Like most religions, The Religion of Thinness has a set of initiation rites. These are things we learn and do to become part of the network of women devoted to trimming and slimming. We may not be conscious of having joined The Community of Thinness or of having agreed to the initiation rites themselves, as they are relatively informal and often involve a gradual training process rather than a singular event. One college student explained:

> I never used to worry about my weight or eating until I came to college. All the other girls were talking about it. I mean *constantly*. And not just in the cafeteria, but throughout the day. It didn't take long for me to start counting calories at every meal and weighing myself whenever I could.

Initiation rites often revolve around being taught some kind of "special" knowledge. This is particularly true in traditional religious and tribal communities where the process of being initiated into a community can be more pronounced than it is in their secular counterparts. The knowledge acquired divides those that have been fully adopted by the community from those who are on the outside. It ensures their status as insiders and this fosters feelings of belonging.

A classic example is the Rite of Communion in the Roman Catholic Church. Catholics aren't allowed to ingest the Eucharist until they reach a certain age (usually around seven or eight). They then go through a ritualized form of education called Catechism. Only after completing this training are they allowed to make their First Communion, during which they receive the Eucharist for the first time. When they do, this rite of passage is honored and observed by other members of the congregation who welcome the new communicant as an "insider," a member of the "body of Christ."

Although The Community of Thinness is not an institutional religion like the Roman Catholic Church, its method of initiation entails a similar educational process. Gaining the "knowledge" necessary to get or stay thin is an important part of a girl's socialization in our culture because it allows her to fit in with her peers. The young woman quoted above learned the caloric content of foods in order to feel accepted by her college friends, who were already active participants in The Community of Thinness.

Some of the "special knowledge" needed to belong to this community includes:

- How many calories, fat grams, and/or carbohydrates in every kind of food

- Who are the most "beautiful" models and actresses and how they stay thin

- How to maximize a workout to burn the most calories

- How to curb cravings with substances like aspartame, saccharin, and nicotine

- What techniques work for restricting eating or purging

- What to wear to look thinner

- How to style your hair to slenderize your face

- Why food is a source of danger (not pleasure)

- Why your body is NOT okay just as it is

Note that this list differs from—though is related to—The Thin Commandments we explored in the last chapter. Here the emphasis is on the acquisition of special concepts, "facts," and techniques through which you secure and demonstrate your membership in The Community of Thinness. Whether or not you are "good" or "bad" in the application of these techniques is less important than knowing the crucial information. As long as you are committed to acquiring such knowledge, you don't risk exclusion.

Many of us didn't have to wait until college for our initiation; our mothers, family members, or friends introduced us to The Community of Thinness at even earlier ages. Some of us were taken to a weight loss meeting as a child, sent to fat camp, or put on a diet under the tutelage of coaches or doctors. And none of us could avoid the media, which taught us almost everything we needed to know to be an insider.

Whatever the case, acquiring this special knowledge elevates your status. It connects you. It makes you belong. A woman who started dieting when she was eight years old recalls:

> I remember how pleased I was the first time my mother instruct-
> ed me about the importance of counting calories. She noted the
> number of calories in a piece of celery compared to a chocolate
> chip cookie. It seems silly now, but at the time I thought she was
> giving me the most important information in the world, and I
> knew intuitively that somehow this knowledge made me closer
> to her, that it meant I was becoming a woman.

Our attraction to The Community of Thinness reveals our longing
to be loved and accepted. Whether the people we turn to for affirmation are as anonymous as Internet bloggers or as close to us as our own
mother, we sense that our chances for getting this love increase greatly
if we learn what they know and share their aspirations to be thinner.
However, while this special knowledge gives us a feeling of being
included, it does so by creating a boundary that can come back to
haunt us when we don't live up to its standards. "Even though I loved
the closeness I felt with my mother because of our shared passion for
thinness," the woman above continued, "it came with strings attached.
I always felt that she loved me more when I was thinner, and that I
risked losing that love by gaining weight."

You may or may not risk losing your mother's love if you gain a few
pounds. But many of us believe—and rightly so, in some cases—that
the approval of others is tied to our external appearance. Do you have
friends, family members, or peers who would disapprove if you refused
to discuss or act on the special knowledge you have acquired through
The Community of Thinness? What would your sister say if you
suggested that she was buying into a false paradigm of beauty every
time she said, "I'm fat"? What would your mother say if you told her
you refused to worry about your weight anymore? Would your best
friend believe you if you told her she is beautiful just as she is? Would
you believe her if she said it to *you?*

Sharing a Common Language: Decoding Our Fat-Talk

As with other religions, our initiation into The Religion of Thinness
involves learning and using the vocabulary familiar to other members

of the community. Without realizing it, many of us grow to rely on this coded language to communicate with each other. For example, "I feel fat" is one of the most commonly-used phrases among girls and women who struggle with body image. To someone outside The Community of Thinness, it doesn't make sense. For one thing, a lot of us who say we "feel fat" are not large-bodied. For another, *fat* is not a *feeling*. It's a judgment—one that is based on comparing yourself to others or to some external ideal you have internalized.

Yet among insiders, the symbolic meaning of this statement is quite clear. It's an expression of anxiety that focuses on the body, yet carries broader meanings. According to Mimi Nichter and Nancy Vuckovic, anthropologists who studied the "fat talk" of female adolescents, girls use such language as a way of saying "I'm not perfect" in the hopes that others will want to include them in their group.[2] But they also use it as an idiom of distress and a call for support.

Given these unspoken meanings, it's not surprising that we often respond to a woman who insists she's "too fat" by identifying with her struggle and by assuring her that it's not true: "What do you mean? You shouldn't worry—you look *great!* I'd give anything to have your body instead of mine." Rather than challenge the paradigm on which The Religion of Thinness is built, such comments reinforce it. By reassuring a woman that she isn't too fat, we implicitly support the idea that there *is* a state of being "too fat" and that it's something we should avoid at all costs. By telling her she has nothing to worry about because she's already thin, we indirectly affirm the importance of being slender, rather than open a critical dialog about where her anxieties come from in the first place and how they might be resolved.

Perhaps we give such assurances to others because we want to receive them ourselves. Or maybe it's just an unconscious habitual response—just one of those things we say—instead of a clearly thought-out statement. In any case, by saying "I feel fat" we are saying much more than how we feel about the size of our bodies. We are asking that others accept us as we are, especially when we have a hard time doing so ourselves. In this seemingly simple, innocent way, we seek to be unconditionally loved.

Food and body are seemingly safe topics that women use to bond with other women. Fat talk often covers anxieties we may not feel comfortable sharing directly. It frees us from the vulnerability we experience when we're open and honest about our real problems. It's a lot easier to talk about weight and calories than our feelings of anxiety or depression, the trouble we're having in our relationships, that our kids are driving us crazy, or that even at our age, we still don't know what we want to do with our lives. Divulging our latest dieting dilemma is socially acceptable, if not encouraged. Our talk about thinness allows us to experience a form of connection and acceptance without requiring us to truly let down our guard. Unfortunately the price we pay for this "safe" way of bonding is that our relationships are often superficial. As such, they cannot give us the basic love and nurturing we truly need.

Confessing our "Sins" in Search of Forgiveness

Another way we reinforce our bonds with others in The Community of Thinness is through the confessions we make about our food and body "failures."

"I ate way too much," we say regretfully as we push our chairs away from the table. Or, "Last night I blew it at Baskin Robbins," or "I'm tempted to skip exercising today." At first glance, these confessions may seem like good ways to unburden ourselves of the discomfort we feel about weight and eating. But much like fat talk, such heartfelt disclosures mask our needs for love and acceptance that The Community of Thinness cannot fulfill.

Informal divulgences of our food and body "weaknesses" mirror the more formal confessions of some Christians, who seek to resolve their pain by admitting their failures to another. In the Catholic Church the practice of confession is considered a sacrament—a rite through which the divine becomes present in a person's attempt to heal. Catholicism teaches that confessing sins to a priest opens the heart to God and thereby to the experience of divine forgiveness, which in turn inspires us to do things differently.

Forgiveness is an integral part of our mental and spiritual health, and relationships play a crucial role in bringing it about. Feeling forgiven is necessary not so much because we have "sinned," but because the self-acceptance we need blossoms when we experience the unwavering acceptance of others.

This need for forgiveness and mutual support is apparent outside the church as well. In different ways, modern-day "confessionals," from self-help groups like Overeaters Anonymous, to psychotherapy, or even daytime talk shows, illustrate the power of talking openly about our problems within a community. Part of what makes experiences like these so compelling is that, to varying degrees, they liberate us from one of the most painful parts of being human: the paralyzing secrecy surrounding our weaknesses. Admitting our shortcomings to others can give us a tremendous sense of relief. By sharing our problems we lessen the burden we feel of trying to carry them ourselves. We also find healing when we learn that someone else is able to identify with our pain, which makes us feel less alone.

The disclosures we make about our weight-loss failures reveal a similar desire for acceptance. By confessing, we seek relief from our shame, and hope that others will love and forgive us despite our weaknesses. A woman confessed at a meeting sponsored by her weight-loss program:

> I don't know what got into me. I was doing really, really well the past few days—staying under my point limit and everything. Then last night I just lost it. It started with just a few bites of my daughter's leftover birthday cake when I was alone cleaning up after the party, and before I knew it, I had eaten three more pieces. I know I just have to start over again and get back on the plan tomorrow. But right now I feel like a total failure.

Sharing the pain of such an episode *could* have the potential to help us let it go. But in the context of The Community of Thinness, such confessions reinforce the notion that there's something wrong with us, that we are indeed failures because we lack self-control, that our problems are rooted in our personal flaws. Without seeing both the social influences on our struggles and the deeper spiritual needs they reveal, we can simply go on believing that losing weight is the answer to our problems. And we'll find plenty of support for this belief among other members of The Community of Thinness.

To forgive is to let go of judgment—both of ourselves and of others. This requires us to soften our hearts and be present to our hurt so that it can be transformed. That means becoming vulnerable and facing up to whatever we have done or whatever was done to us. Doing so allows us to open ourselves up and feel compassion in the midst of suffering. Forgiving others enables us to grow from experiences that have hurt us and frees us to move on. Feeling forgiven allows us to know that we are loved, *regardless*. No matter how horrible we feel about ourselves. No matter how "good" or "bad" we are.

Confessing our weight loss failures to fellow members of The Community of Thinness may give us a temporary glimpse of the love and acceptance we so desperately need. But in the long run it only serves to tie us more tightly to the entire paradigm that is generating our pain in the first place. Such confessions keep us from making the kind of disclosure that would set us on a path of recovering our health and sanity: that our devotion to thinness is making us miserable.

Although, like our fat talk, our expressions of guilt about what we eat *seem* to come from a place of vulnerability, they too are spoken from behind a veil. Saying "I ate way too much" is a way to camouflage the deeper burdens we carry—whether in our relationship to food and our body or in other areas of our life. If we could bravely own and share our lives with people we trust, we might experience the love and acceptance we really need—both from ourselves and others. What's more, we might even discover that we are not alone in our struggle to heal. We might find companions who share our desire for a life much fuller than The Religion of Thinness can give us.

This is a big risk to take. Understandably, many of us fear rejection, even from those closest to us, if we pull back the curtain. And there is no guarantee that people will accept us if we truly open up.

Tragically, these fears can keep us invested in The Community of Thinness, where we know we will be welcomed as long as we follow the rules, speak the language, and confess the "truths" that ensure our inclusion.

Unfortunately, when a community is based on conformity, there is little chance of being accepted—much less forgiven—just as you are. Instead you must strive to be like the other members of the group if you don't want to be left out in the cold.

When Community is Based on Conformity: The End of Self-Acceptance

Alongside our craving to be accepted is the fear of rejection: that horrible feeling of not fitting in. The Religion of Thinness admits anyone into its community with one simple condition: that we strive to be slender. Conformity is the hallmark of faith in The Religion of Thinness, not just in body size, but also in worldview: every woman should want and try to be thinner, regardless of age, ethnicity, sexual orientation, economic status, or creed. As long as she does, she is accepted. And if she doesn't, she'd better find new friends.

Though many of us, including women of African, Hispanic, Jewish, Mediterranean, and Eastern European descent, come from families and cultures that appreciate more ample-bodied women, we are still not immune to the wider social pressure to lose weight. Whatever our hereditary disposition or ethnic heritage, we gravitate to the thin ideal because we want to feel included. And in a society wracked with prejudices of all kinds, trying to "fit in" can come with a heavy price, especially for minority women. A young Hispanic woman recalls the pain of this effort: though she was short for her age, she had never thought of herself as fat, until one day in 7th grade one of her friends suggested she go on a diet:

> As one of two Latina girls at a virtually all-white high school I almost went crazy trying to fit in with my peers. So I bought a pair of sleek designer jeans, and told myself I wasn't going to

eat until I fit into them. My body's always been sort of short and round, like my mother's, my aunts', and my sisters'. I'm still waiting to wear those jeans. It's been 15 years and I'm still waiting.

This woman's experience echoes the findings from a survey in *Essence* magazine, whose mostly black respondents showed high levels of weight preoccupation and disordered eating. The vast majority of those surveyed said they were worried about becoming fat, and many of them attributed their anxiety to their attempts to assimilate into a predominantly white culture that worships thinness. "When I first started practicing bulimic behavior," one of the respondents explained, "I was very much influenced by white beauty standards.... People treat you better when you lose weight and look beautiful."[3]

Tragically, quantitative studies indicate that a growing number of African American, Hispanic, Native American, and Asian women struggle with food and body issues, and qualitative research supports these findings. In her interviews with women who were ethnically, religiously, economically, and sexually diverse, Becky Thompson found that the stresses of acculturation, including the pressures to conform, were a major factor in the development of eating problems.[4]

Like their white counterparts, ethnically diverse women also face media images that promote an unrepresentative standard of thinness. Consider the following magazine advertisement, which offers a compelling example of how The Religion of Thinness only allows for one very narrow standard of beauty—regardless of what traditional cultural norms and expectations may be:

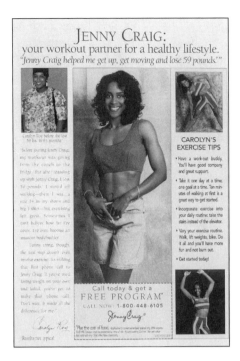

Jenny Craig advertisement

Notice the small picture of Carolyn *before* her seemingly-miraculous weight loss. In this photo she clearly has a full figure. The larger *after* photo of her new, tightly-toned body represents the ideal you can achieve if you become a member of the Jenny Craig community. The ad assumes that you would much prefer to be the thinly-sculpted Carolyn than the full-figured one. Ironically, however, many traditional communities in Africa would view Carolyn's "before" photo as the more beautiful and healthy of the two.

Some women of color start dieting not just because they want to fit in with their European American peers, but also because they reject the stereotypes through which white culture frequently sees them. In her essay, "Fat is a Black Woman's Issue," Retha Powers describes how white cultural norms for female thinness shaped her experiences as a young black girl growing up in a predominantly white neighborhood, where kids called her "Fat Alberta":

> All of the girls who were considered pretty were ultra thin and white, and I was still teased for being ugly. Although now I realize that the ugliness my peers saw had more to do with the darkness of my skin, I reasoned then that I hadn't lost enough weight.[5]

Encouraged by the "Aryan-like" fashion models she studied with her friends while attending a mostly-white high school, Powers went on a diet that later turned into bulimia. When she sought help at the school's counseling office, she was told not to worry about feeling unattractive because "fat is more acceptable in the black community." Then, they invited her to become a "junior counselor" because she was "so stable and could be of help to students with more serious problems."[6]

The desire for acceptance and the pressure to fit in can be especially strong for women whose bodies do not conform to the dominant culture's image of womanhood: the young, white, bourgeois, heterosexual ideal. Like women of color, older, poor, and lesbian women may try to lose weight as a strategy for downplaying their "differences." A woman who had known she was gay since childhood recalled her plan to diet her way into normalcy:

> It was hard enough for my family to accept that I'm gay, the least I could do was try to be skinny. Even if I couldn't *be* a certain way, I was determined to *look* that way.

A woman in her 50s described a parallel struggle to conform her body to a more youthful ideal:

> I don't accept what's happening to my body, especially my figure. The grey hair I can easily color, and a little make-up hides most of the wrinkles. But what about my buttocks and belly? They seem to be forever expanding—no matter how much I exercise, no matter how little I eat! I'd like to know how I'm supposed to love a body like this.

As writer Marjory Nelson observes, "old women" are similar to "fat women" in our culture because both are viewed as "distortions of nature," or "diseased." This view opens the door for a variety of doctors and industries to profit from these women's "problems."[7] Whether we throw money at eye creams, surgery, or diet books, in the end we cannot stop the natural process of growing older, softer, and possibly wider. Ultimately, the energy we spend trying to make our bodies "acceptable" reveals not just how much we yearn to be loved, but also how much we long to love ourselves.

When Community Is Built on Competition: The End of Supportive Relationships

Competition among women is one of the most heart-breaking aspects of The Religion of Thinness, because it distorts our need to connect into a drive to outdo. This spirit of competition creates rivals where we might otherwise have friends and promotes self-hatred where we might otherwise find self-love. When we realize this, the whole concept of a Community of Thinness becomes obviously preposterous and quite sad.

Writer Pamela Houston aptly captures the spirit bred by The Religion of Thinness:

> I am walking down the street in Manhattan, Fifth Avenue in the lower sixties, women with shopping bags on all sides. I realize with some horror that for the last 15 blocks I have been counting how many women have better and how many women have worse figures than I do. Did I say 15 blocks? I meant 15 years.[8]

Potentially supportive relationships lack stability when they are built upon rivalry. While we may enjoy the communal feeling at a gym—chatting and working out with other women—this enjoyment easily sours when we feel jealous of those who look "better" than we do. Discussing our food plan with others at a weight-loss program may come as a relief to us, but this feeling easily gives way to anxiety when we envy those who lose more than we do. Relationships that involve competition may give us a fleeting sense of connection. "At least we're all in this together," we may think. But in the end it's hard to count on a friend who is also an opponent.

What's more, this dimension of The Religion of Thinness helps us avoid, rather than deal with, the underlying insecurities that drive our problems in the first place. We compensate for feeling inadequate or weak by trying to be better than those around us. We ignore the fear of rejection that simmers beneath our jealousy by gossiping about those we feel are a threat.

Instead of helping us explore and work through these uncomfortable feelings directly, relationships based on body size and weight-loss exacerbate them. More often than not, the unspoken contest to see who can be the thinnest is more cutthroat than playful. Our "success" is defined by another's "failure." We feel secretly happy when she gains weight, and silently rivaled when she loses.

Often we don't even know the women we dislike or resent because they are skinny. All we need to know is that they are winning a game we feel compelled to play. Consider what this person said about her husband's coworker:

> When I first met my husband's new colleague, I felt my heart sink to my feet. She was young, blond, pretty, and thin—all the things I wish I could be. I knew right then and there that I didn't like her, and I wished she would be fired or just quit. My husband and I are happily married. But every time he mentions her I get a sick feeling in my stomach.

What does it do to our self-perception when we jump to conclusions about another woman because she is—or isn't—thinner than we are? How can we hope to build the kind of relationships we crave and deserve when our automatic response to is to see someone as a potential barrier to our own happiness?

A lot of us are not conscious of our investment in the "Who's

Thinner?" contest because the competition that fuels it is part of the very air we breathe. An aggressive spirit permeates our culture, which is constantly encouraging us to get ahead. Although rivalry among women is not confined to the pursuit of thinness, it frequently centers on physical appearance, as suggested by the following magazine spread for Pond's anti-aging skin cream:

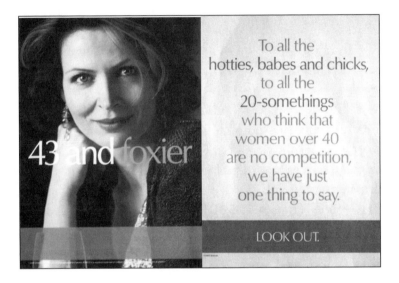

Pond's Anti-Aging Cream advertisement

The pink-lettered copy reads: "To all the hotties, babes, and chicks, to all the 20-somethings who think that women over 40 are no competition, we have just one thing to say. LOOK OUT." The opposite page features a youthful-looking woman—no grey hair or wrinkles, and a flawlessly airbrushed complexion—with the words: "43 and foxier." To women in their 20s, the ad poses a kind of challenge, warning them not to take their youthful advantage for granted. For women over 40, the ad appeals to a sense of adventure: the possibility of accomplishing something against the odds—of becoming "foxier" despite the aging process. In either case, the message is clear: women are connected to each other, but the bond is one of contention.

Yet, somewhere in our hearts, we know that happiness doesn't come from getting ahead. Our life experiences tell us that it's through relationship with others—family, friends, co-workers, religious communities, and, on occasion, even strangers—that we come to experience genuine contentment. "It is in giving that we receive," as the Prayer of St. Francis reminds us. Even the world's most scientific minds acknowledge that we are fundamentally connected and that our separateness is an illusion. Albert Einstein called this sense of separateness a "delusion of consciousness" which imprisons us in self-interests and worries. In his own words, "Our task must be to free ourselves from this prison by widening the circle of understanding and compassion to embrace all living creatures and the whole of nature in its beauty."[9]

This call to connect is profoundly different from the call to confess, conform, and compete sponsored by The Community of Thinness. It encourages us to look beyond self-centered interests and become part of something greater than ourselves. It invites us to accept the parts of ourselves that are vulnerable or tender and share them with those we care about in a mutual attempt to heal. If we can hear the wisdom of this call, we have a real opportunity to find the authentic support we were looking for when we became part of The Community of Thinness.

The Power of Genuine Community: Building Nourishing Relationships

Positive relationships call on us to grow beyond ourselves by expanding our consciousness and opening our hearts. As they do, they relieve us of the burden of our self-seeking egos. Communities that foster our genuine well-being remind us of what we most value. They also nourish our efforts to pursue our larger calling in life. Knowing there are people we can count on to accept us as we are not only allows us to more easily accept ourselves, but it also frees us to take risks, be creative, and engage in the process of self discovery and healing. At the same time, knowing there are people who depend on us can bolster our courage when we feel fearful. The medieval Christian mystic Meister

Eckhart (c. 1260–c. 1328) wrote, "If I were alone in a desert and feeling afraid, I would want a child to be with me. For then my fear would disappear and I would be made strong."[10]

The beauty of healthy connections is that they enable us to rise above our fears and find the strength that is already in us.

But being a member of a community isn't always easy. Relationships bring out the best *and* the worst in us. They remind us of our inner strengths while at the same time they expose our weaknesses. The Indian philosopher J. Krishnamurti (1895–1986) teaches that, "Relationship is the mirror in which we see ourselves as we really are."[11] Perhaps this is why many of us devote ourselves to food and thinness—we fear the vulnerability required in the development of authentic relationships. Yet, we need such connections to keep us honest. It is difficult to be truthful with ourselves about our struggles—as well as our desire to transform them—when we cannot or do not share them with someone.

We may feel a little crazy—and a little lonely—if no one in our family or circle of friends recognizes the insanity of our culture's devotion to thinness. To maintain our health, we need companions who share our alternative mindset and vision. They should be people who consciously refuse to play the game of out-doing each other in the quest for thinness, and who are looking for deeper meaning in their lives. A recovering woman in her late 20s describes her support system:

> My eating disorder started in college when I was surrounded by girls who couldn't stop talking about calories. Thank God I've outgrown those relationships. These days, a lot of my close friends have struggled to some extent with body image and eating issues. But instead of encouraging each other to be thinner, we try to support each other in accepting our bodies and eating healthy. It's nice to have someone to talk to when I see an advertisement that really pisses me off.

We may not already have the kind of relationships that support critical awareness and encourage mindful self-acceptance. But developing and nurturing such connections is a vital part of the journey. There is a Buddhist saying, "If a tiger comes down from its mountain and goes to the valley, people will catch and kill it." It means that if a spiritual seeker leaves the support of her or his community, it becomes difficult to continue practicing.[12] In the same way, learning to love our bodies is not something we can do by ourselves. We need the strength, wisdom, and the example of others who share our desire for personal and social transformation.

The kind of alternative communities we find is less important than the quality of relationships they offer. Some of us may rely primarily on established connections, like friends or family, to help us find our way. Others will benefit from more formal systems, like an eating disorders support group. The key is to forge bonds that stimulate your critical awareness, encourage you to own up to your problems, and provide the love and acceptance you need. The following are a few ideas on ways to find or build communities that can help support you in your journey of healing.

Building a Mindful Community of Critical Thinkers

One possibility is to be proactive in your pursuit of a healthy community by organizing friends, family members, and others who may be drawn to the practices of mindfulness and cultural critique as tools for personal growth.

The benefits of such a community cannot be understated. Imagine the power of sitting silently together with others who seek to become more present to their bodies, their lives, and the world around them. It's not hard to envision the transformative potential of critically analyzing various aspects of The Religion of Thinness (e.g., images, myths, rituals, morality, etc.) with others who seek to deprogram their minds, bodies, and spirits from its destructive influence.

I realize that starting what you might call a "Mindful Community of Critical Thinkers" may sound like a pie-in-the-sky idea. But it doesn't have to be. Of course, it will take both effort and courage on your part, but the rewards you'll find will be well worth it. And you don't have to wait until you are "far enough along" in your healing process to create such a community. You simply need the willingness to try, along with a few ideas about how your group might practice together. Here are some suggestions to get you started.

Recruit Members

Begin by discussing the idea with family members and friends you think would be interested in creating such a community. Certainly many of them are devotees of The Religion of Thinness, and an open invitation to join a group like this may help raise their consciousness and identify with mutual struggles they have had.

As you consider whom to invite to participate, you will need to exercise some caution. Obviously, it's not going to be helpful to have members in the group who are still committed to The Religion of Thinness or who insist on discussing their latest weight-loss triumphs and failures. You may want to widen the circle of people you invite to include colleagues, acquaintances, and schoolmates. You could even hang up flyers to recruit members. I encourage you to be open to anyone you think would be interested in practicing mindfulness and cultural critique as strategies for developing a healthier relationship to food and their bodies.

Use the First Meeting to Establish a Structure

Once you have identified a group of people who want to participate, even if it is as few as two or three, establish an initial meeting time and place. A close-knit group could meet at someone's home, or if there's going to be a wider membership, you can use a community center or classroom.

Though it isn't absolutely necessary, I recommend creating a structure for your meetings. Bring an agenda to the first gathering that lays out some basic ground rules (i.e., the group is *not* a weight-loss club and talk of calories or diets is verboten). The agenda should also address logistical issues to be discussed among participants (i.e., how long the meetings will last, who will facilitate them, how often you plan to meet, etc.). The group will be most effective if you can meet weekly for at least an hour, but if this sounds daunting, a couple of hours monthly are a good start. At your initial gathering, you should also consider how much time during each meeting you want to devote to mindfulness practice and how much to cultural criticism. Details can be worked out later, but establishing a general framework will be helpful.

Whether or not you decide to have a regular facilitator for future meetings, you will need to fill that role to get things started. At the first meeting, thank people for coming and share your own reasons for forming the group. Then have everyone take turns introducing themselves (if necessary) and expressing their goals for participating. I suggest keeping this portion of the program relatively brief; this is not the time for anyone to monopolize the discussion. One of your tasks is to keep the group focused and on schedule. Once everyone's had a chance to speak, you are ready to move to the heart of the meeting.

Introduce the Practices of Mindfulness and Cultural Critique

This is where you can introduce the concepts of mindfulness and cultural critique. For mindfulness, you might guide the group through the "Sitting Still and Watching Your Breath" exercise in Chapter 1. (I suggest reviewing this before the meeting to prepare.) You can use other exercises from this book at future meetings. For the cultural critique portion, choose another experiential activity. For instance, you could bring an example of popular culture (e.g., a magazine ad or article, a film, news report, book, etc.) that promotes The Religion of Thinness, and deconstruct its message with everyone's help.

As homework, members might collect other media examples to critique at your next meeting. Or, the group might read and discuss chapters from this book. Whatever you choose, try to involve everyone in more ways than just talking by including participatory activities such as sitting and breathing mindfully and critically examining aspects of popular culture that support The Religion of Thinness.

Concluding the Meeting

Before the end of the first meeting, be sure to establish the following:

- When and where the next meetings will be

- Who will plan the agendas

- What kinds of activities will be included

- Whether or not to recruit additional members

- What homework needs to be done

In order to end on a positive note and promote a sense of community, try to bring everyone together in some way as you close the meeting. You might spend the last five minutes sitting together in silence, sending thoughts of peace, respect, and acceptance to yourself and each other, and concluding with the sound of a bell. Or, you could invite each person to offer aloud a wish they have for the other members, using phrases like "May you be _____," or "May you feel _____" (i.e., courageous, healthy, serene, etc.). Another possibility would be to ask everyone to share an intention they have for practicing peace with their bodies during the upcoming week. This kind of closing ritual fosters a sense of connection within the group and strengthens each individual's commitment to pursue this path of healing together.

The Challenges and Rewards of Communal Practice

If you are consistent in your practice together, you will find that eventually the group takes on a life of its own, and the process will fall into place. The benefit of maintaining some kind of structure is that it keeps the group focused on the practices themselves (i.e., mindfulness and cultural critique) rather than the personalities or specific problems of individual members.

Of course, some challenges are bound to arise. There will be times, for example, during conversations when people veer off topic, can't sit still and listen, or when they become argumentative. Disagreements can be uncomfortable, but they can also be opportunities for growth if explored in an atmosphere of respect. If discussions get out of control, it may be helpful to use a "talking stick" that gets passed around so that only one person speaks at a time.

There is not one "right" way to handle the challenges that will inevitably arise in the context of your new community. When they happen, try to find ways for the group to gently remind each other of the purpose of the practices you are engaged in and the personal growth you mutually seek. Being part of a community is a dynamic experience and the structure shouldn't be so rigid as to allow for no flexibility. Stay open to the people in the group as you stay focused on your intent and you will see that your mindfulness practice and your skills in cultural critique will develop and flourish—individually *and* together.

I understand that you might be skeptical of starting such a group. But it really is a viable option. As part of her recovery from compulsive eating, a woman in her 50s started a women's support group by inviting a few friends to meet twice a month. She encouraged each of them to bring a friend who shared an interest in midlife self-discovery. Within a short time, a group of eight women was regularly gathering in each other's living rooms, entrusting each other with their struggles, insecurities, and aspirations. Though not all of them had experienced eating problems, troubled body image was a recurrent theme. The woman who started the group described its impact:

> Even the women who had never had an eating disorder talked about being unhappy with their bodies. After all those years of feeling alone in my struggles, this revelation was very healing. The other women's willingness to be vulnerable about their own problems is giving me the self-acceptance and strength I need to continue moving forward in my own recovery.

You can have a similar experience. Your choice to create a Mindful Community of Critical Thinkers will strengthen your capacity to love and respect yourself and others in ways you might not anticipate and certainly won't experience if you don't try.

But if for some reason you do not feel drawn to organize a group, there are other alternatives.

Other Self-Help Group Alternatives to
The Religion of Thinness

Many people who suffer from eating problems find loving support for their recovery in the 12-step group, Overeaters Anonymous (OA). Unlike commercial weight-loss programs, this organization is nonprofit and is not focused on thinness. Instead, OA emphasizes overall well-being, including spiritual health, as the goal of healing from eating problems. Men and women congregate at meetings, laughing and crying together as they tell their stories and explore the spiritual malaise behind their unwanted eating patterns. The fluid structure of meetings (leadership is rotating) and the give-what-you-can price of admission (a voluntary collection is taken at each meeting) make OA a nonhierarchical and noncommercial forum for personal change.

In OA, people discover they are not alone in their food and body prisons. Some of the "tools" for recovery advocated by this program—making phone calls, having a sponsor, working the steps, keeping a journal, going to meetings, helping others—not only foster more mindful eating behavior but also more honest relationships with oneself and others. By using such tools, countless OA members have experienced relief from the secrecy that contributes to their isolation and shame. Although the spirituality of OA fails to explicitly incorporate a critique of our culture's obsession with thinness, it seems perfectly possible to weave the kind of social criticism offered in this book into this communally-oriented recovery program.

Some of us, however, may prefer groups that are more intentional about maintaining the link between spirituality and cultural criticism. A growing number of such groups is emerging around the country. Though their methods vary, many use "consciousness raising" as a means for cultivating self-understanding and for probing life's big questions. By listening to one another's stories—not just problems with body image, but also difficulties with careers, relationships, families, and so forth—participants learn to recognize the societal patterns and cultural expectations that contribute to their common problems. Understanding the social dimensions of our "personal" issues empowers us to move past self-blame and criticism towards a more constructive understanding of our life's purpose.[13] You may be able to find similar groups on college campuses, through alternative newspapers, or on flyers at places like health food stores, yoga centers, and independent bookstores.

Resources from Traditional Religious Communities

While many who are drawn to the kind of communities just described are seeking alternatives to organized religion, some of us are more likely to meet our relational needs through conventional spiritual connections. All of the major religions have spiritual teachings that implicitly call into question The Religion of Thinness. The Jewish and Muslim critique of idolatry, for example—the idea that God alone deserves our devotion—challenges our culture's worship of thinness and the beliefs and behaviors it encourages. The Hindu appreciation of diversity—the belief that one God is manifest in an infinite variety of ways and forms—suggests an alternative to the monotonous, uniform vision of "truth" and "beauty" circulated by popular media images. The Christian doctrine of the Incarnation—that divinity became embodied in the person of Jesus, that God assumed the form of human flesh—suggests the goodness of *every* body, regardless of its size, shape, or color. And the Buddhist teaching of impermanence—the notion that everything changes and nothing lasts forever—exposes the illusion of the security we often seek by believing we can control our lives and bodies.

Those of us who embrace these traditions might consider starting a group that explores these kinds of tenets and their challenges to The Religion of Thinness. In the process, we may uncover additional resources within our particular heritage that lend new meaning to our efforts.

We might also develop a relationship with a mentor to guide our search for wholeness and healing. In recent years, this practice has been on the rise as an increasing number of people seek the wisdom of spiritual directors and gurus in an effort to integrate their sacred values more deeply into their daily life.[14] Through deep, compassionate listening, such advisors help us discern, explore, and ultimately transform our suffering. The word *guru* means "one who is heavy," suggesting that an effective spiritual mentor is so grounded that nothing we say or do could shatter her or his ability to continue loving us and encouraging us to do the difficult work of changing our relationship to food and our bodies. Though building a meaningful bond with a teacher requires a great deal of trust on our part, the relationship should not promote dependence. As Hindu scholar and author Eknath Easwaran (1910–1999) points out, one of the guru's most important tasks is to make us aware of the teacher within ourselves and to increase our access to our own sense of truth.[15]

Whether or not you embark on a formal relationship with a spiritual guide, you are likely to benefit from connecting with people who have successfully traveled the path of recovery. Without the wisdom of seasoned veterans, it is easy to flounder. As the 13th century Sufi mystic poet Rumi observed, "Whoever travels without a guide needs 200 years for a two-day's journey."[16]

Sharing Our Problems Outside a Religious Setting

You may be fortunate enough to have people in your life—family, co-workers, relatives, friends—who are spiritually "heavy" enough to be present to your pain and to listen compassionately to your struggles. But not everyone will be so lucky, and you may need to look beyond the sphere of your current relationships to find people you can count on to love you through the challenges you face, people who are committed to their own spiritual growth and who share your critical awareness of The Religion of Thinness.

This kind of nurturing relationship can often be found with a therapist or other healthcare professional. A growing number of therapists not only offer spiritually sensitive counseling, but are also incorporating cultural critique into their work with clients who have eating problems. Speaking your truth with a skilled guide is an effective way to integrate the various dimensions of recovery. To find someone with expertise in these areas, you may need to do some research and interviewing. Try using some referral sources for an eating disorders specialist or a professional who specializes in mind/body therapy or psychospiritual development.

Whether or not you make formal therapy part of this process, you need relationships that help you become honest about your struggles and encourage you to learn from them. The journey of healing really begins when we find the courage to share our problems with someone who can listen—without judging or trying to fix us. A woman in her 40s, who has been in recovery for over two decades, recalls the transformative effects of telling someone about her eating disorder for the first time:

> I was in college, and I was taking a walk with my boyfriend of almost two years, and though he'd always been very sweet to me, I was terrified of telling him about my bulimia. But something in me knew it was time. I guess it was the part of me that wanted to get better. And so I told him about it. I told him how it started back in junior high, how I lived in fear of someone finding out, and how it was ruining my life. And do you know what? Instead of being all grossed out or telling me what I should do, he stopped walking and put his arms around me. I started to cry. I think telling him made it very real, like I couldn't pretend anymore. I knew that being honest with him meant I would finally have to stop lying to myself.

Taking the risk to talk about your eating problem may be one of the most difficult things you have ever done or will do. But it is also one of the most loving, because it can unlock the door to your healing.

Organizations and Movements with a Wider Vision

To find companions who will walk with us on our journey, we may look to some of the organizations and movements dedicated to promoting self-acceptance at any size. Some of these are quite intentional in their critique of our culture's obsession with thinness. The National Association to Advance Fat Acceptance (NAAFA) is a human rights organization working to eliminate discrimination based on body size and to empower people through education, advocacy, and support. Founded in 1969, the NAAFA "maxim" is to accept oneself at one's current size, to stay active, and to get on with one's life. Offering brochures such as *Declaration of Health Rights for Fat People* and *Dispelling Myths About Fat People,* this group works to educate both its members and the general public about the facts and fictions regarding the lives of our large-bodied brothers and sisters (*www.naafa.org*).

Additionally, an increasing number of health professionals have adopted the "Health At Every Size" philosophy. This new paradigm offers a compassionate, health-focused alternative to the guilt-inducing, isolating approach traditionally used by the medical establishment. Promoting pleasurable movement and intuitive eating are among the practices they advocate.[17]

There are also numerous groups and movements offering avenues for networking and connecting with others who challenge The Religion of Thinness. The National Eating Disorders Association (NEDA) is the largest not-for-profit organization in the United States dedicated to preventing eating disorders and providing treatment referrals to those who suffer from anorexia, bulimia, binge eating, and body image issues (*www.nationaleatingdisorders.org*). A good place to find more information is Gürze Books, which specializes in eating disorders education and resources—including the development and publication of *The Religion of Thinness*—and has links to about 50 proactive organizations worldwide at their website, *www.gurze.com*.

Reconnecting with Our Cultural Roots

Our ethnic heritage can be another resource for addressing our relational needs, particularly for minority women. Connecting with our cultural roots can be a tremendous source of support because it links us to a community of people whose lives have been shaped by a common history. Instead of trying to assimilate our "difference," we can learn to embrace it in the company of others. Enjoying diversity in all its forms, hues, and sizes is an essential component of self-acceptance.

One diversity-affirming tradition that is threatened by mainstream society's emphasis on thinness is the appreciation of full-figured women in some ethnic communities. For example, in her book *Hungry for More: A Keeping-It-Real Guide for Black Women on Weight and Body Image,* Robyn McGee notes that historically, "African Americans have rejected the skin-and-bones, anorexic, adolescent boy-shaped standard of beauty popular with white women since the Victorian era." According to McGee, "No one wants a bone but a dog" is an old saying in the black community that affirms the value of women with well-rounded bodies. Hispanic culture includes a similar aesthetic. Mexican American Christy Haubegger explains how this sensibility makes it possible for some Latinas to enjoy their God-given beauty:

> People who don't know us may think we're fat. At home, we're called *bien cuidadas* (well cared for). . . Whether we're Cuban American, Mexican American, Puerto Rican, or Dominican, food is a central part of Hispanic culture. . . You feed people you care for, and so if you're well cared for, *bien cuidadas,* you have been fed well.[18]

In addition to retrieving cultural traditions that promote self-acceptance, minority women might come together to critically reflect on the ways racism contributes to their troubled relationships to food and their bodies.[19] The inner doubt and self-loathing experienced by many minorities points to an internalized racism—the unconscious acceptance of racist stereotypes—that leads some to seek solace in weight-loss or eating. In 1998, a longtime member of Overeaters Anonymous, together with her friends, started an off-shoot of this 12-Step Program. "Ebony OA" is a sisterhood that addresses the particular challenges facing African Americans and Hispanics who struggle with food addiction. "I believe internalized racism is at the core of the compulsive overeating in the black community," the founder explained.[20] A safe place to explore this connection is fundamental for minority women's recovery.[21]

Whatever your color or cultural background, becoming mindful of the links between your internal dialogue and the cultural messages you've absorbed enables you to be more selective about the voices you let into your head and more intentional about the attitude you adopt toward your flesh. Cultivating this awareness in the company of others not only gives you the courage you need to love your body; it also kindles the vision you need to help create a society in which all bodies are considered beautiful.

Change Is Possible, If We Work Together

The shifting landscape of gender and race in the United States provides a hopeful example of how seemingly-ingrained social patterns can change as a result of people working together. Less than 100 years ago, women were not allowed to vote. Less than 50 years ago, black women were not permitted to enter the Miss America Pageant.[22] Less than 50 years ago, women were not admitted to some of the country's most prestigious educational institutions, such as Harvard, Columbia, and Dartmouth. Newspaper want ads were divided into "Help Wanted Male" and "Help Wanted Female" sections, with the female side listing positions for secretaries, domestic workers, and other low-wage service jobs.[23] Less than 60 years ago, racial segregation was perfectly legal in parts of U.S. In the South, blacks and whites couldn't eat at the same restaurants or share bathrooms, much less play, study, or work together. The mere idea of a black president was inconceivable. While we have a long way to go before our country becomes a place where citizens of all ethnic backgrounds enjoy equal opportunity and respect, these examples illustrate just how far we have come, and how it is possible to affect social change if we work together.

In the same way, beginning with our own circles of friends, families, co-workers, neighbors, social groups, and religious communities, we can build coalitions that challenge our society's "thin-size-fits-all" mentality. Together, we can insist that all people deserve to live with dignity inside their own bodies, explore the true meaning of their lives, and experience the joy of physical existence. This kind of solidarity allows us to move from conformity to acceptance—both of ourselves and of the magnificent diversity in our world.

7

FROM ESCAPE TO PRESENCE

"The Salvation of Thinness" and Our Need for Peace

Erica took a deep breath and decided to play with the kids instead of helping in the kitchen. This was the kind of family gathering that triggered her urge to eat long after the dishes were cleared from the table. But she was learning that if she recognized and accepted this urge—instead of automatically acting on it or trying to resist it—the feeling would eventually fade. Redirecting her energy into a game of hide-and-seek with her nieces and nephews would help her forget about the leftover pies and cookies that beckoned.

What Erica wanted most was peace. Peace from the family arguments that drew her in so easily. Peace from her mother's comments about her figure. Peace from the battle she had been waging with food and her body. She wanted to stop getting hooked by her desire to please everyone. She wanted to feel whole from within and secure and centered in her own flesh.

Occasionally she still found herself resorting to old patterns of overeating and restricting. But, more and more, she was learning to pause long enough to make a conscious choice to do things differently. Her support group and daily meditation practice were helping.

So, as much as the family dynamics made her want to escape into the leftover desserts, Erica decided that tonight was yet another opportunity to strengthen new habits.

One of the underlying attractions of The Religion of Thinness is that it enables us to avoid, at least for a while, the real difficulties of our lives. When we are drawn into—or fed up with—dysfunctional family dynamics, we can bury ourselves in leftover desserts. When the circumstances of our lives feel overwhelming, we can withdraw into our own little world of fat grams and calories. When we're totally stressed and on the verge of collapse, we can escape into our obsession with weight loss and the fantasy of physical perfection.

Unfortunately, running away creates far more problems than it solves for several reasons.

First, trying to escape from our difficulties instead of facing and dealing with them (or at least learning to accept and live with them) keeps us in a state of denial. This not only stunts our personal growth, but usually creates more pain in the long run.

Second, when we focus on weight and food to distract us from our distress, we add another layer of suffering to the pain we are trying to escape in the first place—the suffering that comes from our inability to accept our bodies as they are.

Third, practicing The Religion of Thinness means that we buy into false hope that if we just lose enough weight, shed those last few pounds, firm up our tummy, fit into our "skinny jeans," we will finally be at peace. We will achieve *The Salvation of Thinness* and our troubles will miraculously vanish. Of course, part of us knows this isn't true. But another part of us clings to the hope that losing weight *will* save us, that somehow it *will* make everything okay.

The trouble with this equation (thinness = salvation) is not only that it's untrue, but also that it keeps the possibility of peace perpetually in the future—when you're "thin enough." As you may have already figured out, there is actually no such thing as "thin enough" in this salvation plan: there will always be a few more pounds to lose, a few less fat grams to consume, a few more calories to burn.

True inner peace is not a blissful state we achieve by eliminating the parts of ourselves that trouble us. It is not a place we can escape to by getting rid of our unwanted thoughts and feelings. Instead, it is born as we become aware and inquisitive of these aspects of our experience so that we can learn from them. Peace develops when, instead of running, we become present to the full reality of our lives, including the situations and feelings that scare us or make us suffer. Peace comes when we *stop* trying to escape.

How then *do* we deal with the hard times in our life? If running away only increases our pain, how can we learn to be and stay present? How can we accept our compulsion to eat, starve, count or burn calories without acting on those impulses? How can we be peaceful with our bodies and our lives just as they are?

Although I certainly don't have all the answers, years of critiquing The Religion of Thinness have taught me a few things about the path to peace, that I will share:

- **The peace we seek is already within us.** It's not something outside ourselves. We won't experience peace in some distant future (when we have a "better" body). We will only come in contact with it here and now, in our bodies, in our present life situation, in the present moment.

- **The very problems we are trying to escape contain the opportunities we need to grow.** Transforming our problems into occasions for spiritual growth is a vital part of our healing journey. No matter how much pain disordered eating has caused, it contains an opportunity for awakening to a deeper sense of meaning and fulfillment in life. It is a chance to discover or rediscover what is really important and to act on that.

- **Practicing acceptance with our bodies helps us to live in the moment.** Each time we take a deep breath and decide to think and act in ways that honor and nourish our bodies, we water the seeds of peace inside us, enabling them to grow. In so doing, we reconnect to the physical ground of our existence and free ourselves to be fully present here and now.

- **The more we practice peace with our bodies, the more peace we experience in our lives.** There's a strong relationship between how we relate to our bodies and how we relate to life. When we give our bodies the nourishment they need, enjoy the strength they possess, approach them with respect, gratitude, and trust, and accept them as they are, rather than resist or try to "fix" them, we learn how to encounter the world in the same spirit. This brings peace to ourselves and everyone around us.

- **Peace is *the journey* towards greater well-being; it is not the goal.** Peace is a practice, not a destination—a process not a product. It is a path that you walk every moment of your life as you strive to live according to your inner wisdom and in the light of your ultimate purpose.

The "Good Health" of Salvation: Ending Our Battle with Our Bodies

For those of us who grew up thinking that salvation is a reward we get when we die and go to heaven, the etymology of the term "salvation" may be surprising. It is related to the Latin word, *salve*, which means "good health." In this sense, to be saved is to experience wholeness and well-being, what we might consider as peace of mind, body, and spirit. In the context of healing from our disordered relationship to food and our bodies, this definition of salvation is quite revealing.

As we have seen, The Religion of Thinness implicitly promises us The Salvation of Thinness—health, happiness, and a life without problems—if we can achieve some imagined state of physical perfection. However, we know that "good health" entails much more than having a particular kind of body. It encompasses mental, emotional, physical, and spiritual well-being, which are qualities that no amount of weight loss can provide. If we can let go of the assumption that health and thinness are somehow equated, we free ourselves to see salvation from a much broader perspective, namely, as the holistic pursuit of a life full of meaning, presence, and peace.

This approach is found in some Native American traditions in which good health involves belief and trust in a creative life power, a spiritual presence that animates the universe and each individual body within it. Because the Spirit of life pervades every part of existence, including those aspects of ourselves we find unappealing, *everything* is potentially sacred.

From this integrative perspective, "good health" is defined not as a physical state of perfection but as an attitude towards life. Thus, even a woman who is dying, diseased, or disabled can be said to be in good health, if, with the support of her community, she is living her life to the fullest, confronting her difficulties with honesty, integrity, and courage, and trusting the creative power of life.[1]

This perspective is present in other religious traditions as well. The spiritual teachings of Paramahansa Yogananda (1893–1952), a Hindu yogi, stress a similar connection between faith and healing. Yogananda encouraged his readers to use "thought as medicine" by practicing mental affirmations that promote inner peace and physical wellness.[2] He taught that faith in God, cultivated through the responsible use of our own God-given powers, was the key to overall health and harmony.

Jesus of Nazareth, too, practiced a ministry that integrated physical and spiritual well-being. In the gospel of Luke, he instructs his disciples to heal those who are sick and say to them, "the kingdom of God has come near you" (Luke 10:9). When a woman suffering from prolonged menstrual bleeding was instantly healed upon touching his garment, Jesus turned to her and explained that it was her faith that had made her whole (Matthew 9:12).

Each of these examples illustrates the importance of faith in healing. But notice that, in each case, faith is not a set of beliefs, nor is it confined to creeds or defined by doctrine. Rather, faith is an attitude one has towards life and is characterized by a combination of courage and acceptance.

Acceptance and the Peace It Engenders

True peace develops as we learn to accept ourselves, our bodies, and our lives as they are, even as we strive to confront and transform our difficulties with bravery and perseverance.

The idea of accepting your body just as it is contradicts everything you have learned from The Religion of Thinness. The more time you have devoted to this false faith, the more patience, courage, and repeated practice you will need to adopt a new approach. Think of it as a new habit you are cultivating: the habit of acceptance. When you find yourself thinking about how happy you would be if you were thinner, practice acceptance. When you feel the desire to keep eating even though you're no longer physically hungry, or when you want to purge because you think you had "one bite too many," try to stay present. Practice this non-controlling approach whenever you find yourself cringing at the sight of your thighs, or tallying the calories you ate at dinner.

This doesn't mean accepting whatever you are thinking or feeling as "true" and acting on it. On the contrary, it means acknowledging your experience just as it is without placing any judgments on it. Accept that you are *having the thought* that you would be happier if you were thinner, but don't accept the "truth" of the thought. (This same strategy applies to each of the examples given above.) Notice that acceptance here is not about passive resignation, but active awareness. It's about staying present to your experience, as it arises.

I am not asking you to blindly believe in this technique. I am asking you to experiment with a new attitude toward your body and life. See what happens when, instead of resisting or buying into The Religion of Thinness, you consciously allow the thoughts to be there, without acting on them or judging them.

It may sound strange, but accepting yourself just as you are—including outward appearance, internal experience, and life situation—is one of the most effective ways to change your relationship to food and your body. The minute you start accepting things just as they are, you begin to transform your long-standing patterns of abusing your body. What's more, in this holistic model of good health, the very things that make you suffer become opportunities for growth and peace. Ultimately, through the practice of mindful acceptance, you will learn to treat your body as a friend instead of an enemy. This means:

- Being present to (and in) your body

- Listening honestly to what it says

- Responding to its needs with love and care

- Accepting it as it is

- Taking time to enjoy your physicality

These gestures of friendship will improve your health on *every* level—regardless of your particular body shape or size.

Those of us whose physical health might improve if we lost some weight need to beware of the pitfalls of making weight-loss a priority. Dieting our way to "wellness" tends to put us at war with the very bodies we are trying to heal. Our "excess" weight becomes an "enemy" we are trying to eliminate. Even if we succeed in losing weight, we may live in fear of its return. This mentality fosters a state of negativity within us, which diminishes our well-being.

To prioritize weight-loss in our search for peace and wholeness is to put the cart before the horse, because our struggle with weight is often a symptom of an underlying disconnection from our ultimate purpose. However, discovering a more nourishing and meaningful purpose in life and beginning to act on it connects us to an inner strength that will ultimately help us make better choices about eating, exercise, and self-care. And sometimes, weight will come off *as a result*. This is putting the cart firmly *after* the horse, where it belongs.

This broader understanding of health and salvation opens our eyes to an important insight: salvation is the healing and peace we can experience, in our bodies and in the world around us, even *on the journey* toward "good health."

Peace Is Now: Seeing Heaven All Around Us

In fact, the peace we long for is not a distant dream, but an experience that is available this very moment to those who seek it. When Jesus spoke of the "kingdom of heaven," he was not talking about a far-off place in the clouds that we go to when we die. His teachings emphasize the *immediacy* of our connection with the source of well-being: "the kingdom of heaven is in our midst" (Luke 17:21). Peace is not something we earn or receive when we finally achieve the perfect figure or put our disordered eating behind us. We can experience peace *right here and now*—even at times when we feel most stuck.

Practicing loving kindness towards ourselves and others is the key. If we look closely at Jesus' teachings, we see the particular importance of loving those who are vulnerable and scorned: the poor and the sick, the prostitutes and tax collectors, and others whom society typically despises. The message is that true love is *inclusive:* it means loving even the "unlovable." Like good health, real love is holistic.

This teaching on love is instructive not just for relating to others but also to ourselves. To truly love ourselves means to care deeply for *all* our parts, not just those that make us feel confident and successful. For those of us with eating problems, loving what seems unlovable—loving our "enemy"—means loving our bodies as they are. This requires treating them with kindness and respect. A woman who was recovering from years of self-destructive dieting reflected on this process:

> It took me a long time to realize how much my body hatred was hurting me spiritually. My constant berating of it infiltrated the way I saw the rest of the world. Now, I'm working on loving my body. For me, this doesn't mean convincing myself that my body looks great. Maybe I'll get there eventually, but for now

it's just about treating my body with the basic kindness and decency that I would want to show another person. I wouldn't deprive someone of food when they're hungry or torture them with constant criticism just for being who they are. So why do this to myself?

Loving our bodies is not a matter of adoring our appearance. We practice loving our bodies by thinking and behaving in ways that respect and nurture our physicality, rather than trying to subdue or "fix" it. We become present to our physical form, just as it is, and live from within it, mindfully aware of the miracle of life that flows through us and connects us to the wider world.

As Thich Nhat Hanh reminds us: "Our opportunity for peace is not later. It is now."[3]

No matter what you are doing, you always have a choice to treat your body with loving kindness. Even at times when this seems impossible, you can be good to yourself. No matter where you are, what you are doing, or how stressed out, depressed, obsessed, or lost you feel, you can always:

- Slow down and take a refreshing, deep breath.

- Observe your thoughts and the feelings they create and let them drift in and out of your consciousness.

- Bring your attention back to your in-breath and out-breath to help you get present in your body.

- Pay attention to what your body is telling you. Notice the physical sensations within, even if you don't like what you feel.

- Become fully present to your environment and the world around you. See, hear, smell, and touch the things in your surroundings as if for the first time.

- Realize that what is happening "in your head" is little more than a fantasy, a mental movie.

- Go for a walk and be mindful of each step. Remind yourself that the tough times are the best for practicing a loving approach.

This path is not an easy one. But, in each of us, there is a place that is calm and serene, like the bottom of the ocean where the water is quiet and still, even though waves are crashing on the surface. Through our efforts to perfect our bodies, we have neglected this peaceful place inside of us. Now we have a chance to rediscover it by approaching our eating problems with mindful awareness. This is the path of healing.

Rediscovering the peace that is already within you won't make your issues with food and weight miraculously disappear. Nor will it make the pain that led you to develop these issues suddenly evaporate. But being able to touch that peaceful place within you during times of suffering will allow you to feel whole in spite of it. Every time you practice mindfully returning to that tranquil place of acceptance, you increase your capacity to deal with pain and enjoy your life *as it is*.

Suffering is part of the human condition—not an indication that we're doing something wrong. The question is, do we continue trying to avoid our misery and distress by fixating on food or thinness (which, remember, only makes the pain worse), or can we find the courage to be present to these unpleasant feelings, work with them, learn from them, and eventually transform them into wisdom that opens our hearts and enables us to heal ourselves and be present to others?

You may feel so far from that peaceful place inside of you that it's hard to believe you'll ever find your way back to it. Many women who are now recovered once experienced a similar state of hopelessness. But like them, you have the capacity to heal, no matter how distraught or dejected you now feel. At the end of Lindsey Hall's story of recovery from bulimia, she wrote about her journey:

> As weird as it may sound, my bulimia is responsible for who and where I am today, because without such a serious illness I might never have worked so hard to be happy. I had to overcome every barrier that was in my way so that I could live and love fully, with my own set of values and ideals. From eating without fear, I learned to live without fear, and that has truly set me free.[4]

Finding peace is a process that takes time, bravery, and commitment. But instead of encouraging us in this endeavor, our culture pressures us to run away from our problems through an endless array of distractions.

Running Away from Ourselves in a Culture of Distractions

The Salvation of Thinness is part of a larger societal pattern in which we repeatedly look for quick-fixes and external gratifications to divert our attention away from our internal dissatisfaction. An array of distractions compete for our attention, not to mention our money, making it easy to avoid our lives, our problems, and ourselves.

The idea that society provides diversionary tools that keep us from exploring who we truly are is not new. In the 19th century, political theorist Karl Marx (1818–1883) launched his critique of religion, accusing it of being an instrument of denial. He described religion as "the opiate of the masses," because he believed it functioned like a drug, numbing people to their day-to-day struggles and enabling them to deny their suffering and suppress their creativity by fixating their attention on an illusionary, other-worldly goal: heaven. Marx thought that Christianity implicitly taught people to quietly accept or blatantly ignore the actual problems of *this* life.

We need not become Marxists to appreciate the insight of his perspective. The Religion of Thinness *does* function as a present-day "opiate of the masses." Faith in thinness *does* direct our attention away from what's really happening in our lives and the world around us, and fixates our energies on some hoped-for salvation in the future—when we are thinner. What's more, this particular way of evading our problems is both socially acceptable and rewarded. With the blessing of our culture, we exchange "good health" for the short-term pain relief of obsession.

The Religion of Thinness is only one among a myriad of "opiates" our culture provides that numb us to our pain and allow us to escape rather than actively engage with the sources of our struggles. The media, in particular, inundates us with television shows, magazines, advertisements, and films that capture our attention without involving us in self-discovery or social critique, as good art is meant to do. Whether we are watching screaming images of hatred and violence, irresponsible depictions of sexuality, or the happily-ever-after romances that obscure the nature of real relationships, we are generally asked to turn off the critical faculty of our minds.

And, as we have discovered throughout this book, the media we consume does more than entertain. It shapes our understanding of "reality," whether we know it or not. So it's worth asking ourselves what happens when we use it as a means for escaping our problems. How does it affect our psyche—our soul—when, in an attempt to relax and have fun, we watch yet another super-skinny actress engage in one more meaningless relationship with some powerful, hunky man? What happens to our worldview when, in an effort to soothe our anxiety or depression, we flip through page after page of a woman's magazine, absorbing all its schizophrenic messages about food and our figures?

Consider this cover from *Fitness* magazine:

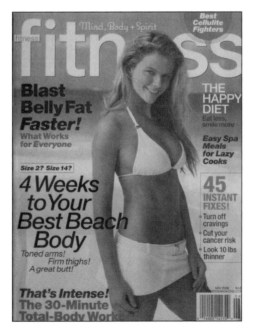

Fitness, May 2008

Unlike publications such as *Vogue* or *Cosmo*, which support The Religion of Thinness with gaunt-faced, anorexic-looking models who inhabit the world of high fashion and hyper-sexuality, *Fitness* belongs to a more recent genre of women's magazines that promote devotion to thinness through the promise of "good health." The assurance of "salvation" in these newer publications is often couched in holistic language. Notice the phrase "Mind, Body and Spirit" just above the magazine title. This vocabulary is particularly seductive for those who consciously seek a deeper, more integrative experience of well-being.

This makes it all-the-more unfortunate and insidious that the vision of good health espoused in publications like *Fitness* is defined almost exclusively through reference to having a "better" (thinner) body. "Size 2? Size 14?" The copy asks—as if it didn't matter. But if it really doesn't make a difference what size you are, then why do almost all of the articles featured on the *Fitness* cover aim to draw you in by promising you a firmer figure? You can "Blast Belly Fat Faster" (and presumably experience peace much sooner). Or you can create "Your Best Beach Body" in just "4 Weeks" (which may not seem like a long time to wait for "salvation," but notice how it's still a future dream). If these strategies don't calm your mind and lift your spirits, there's always the "30 Minute Total Body Workout" or "The Happy Diet" to get you smiling. In fact, there is only one reference (cancer) on the entire cover that is not related to thinness.

As far as I know, no one has ever experienced the peace of mind, body, and spirit that *Fitness* promises by discovering the "Best Cellulite Fighters." This war-like language should clue us into the kind of "good health" the magazine fosters, namely, one that encourages you to go to battle with your body by keeping you on the endless treadmill of physical improvement, while diverting your attention away from the real sources of fulfillment in your life. If you think you are doing yourself a favor by reading *Fitness* magazine (or others like it) because of its purported attention to health and overall well-being, you might want to think again.

How about asking whether the well-being and serenity you are looking for really require you to "look 10 lbs. thinner." And you might ask whether the stereotypical image of the young, blond, happy, thin model, far removed from the cares of the world and enjoying herself on some lovely beach, is what peace of mind, body, and spirit look like *for you.* As soon as you ask these questions, The Salvation of Thinness that this magazine tacitly sponsors starts to look a lot like the empty promise that it is.

Asking such critical questions can be an act of good health, insofar as they lead us back to our inner wisdom. Such questions shift our attention away from the diversionary promise of escape to the reality of our lives unadorned.

One of the reasons our reality may seem unappealing is that we compare it to the "reality" we see on television, online, or in magazines and movies. This media "reality" features an endless litany of luxurious homes, glamorous clothes, expensive cars, and "pretty" (thin) people, whose problems are typically resolved in a happy ending. It's hard not to fantasize about how great our lives would be if we were in their shoes. Given the complications and stresses in our real lives, it doesn't take long before we allow such media fantasies to transport us to a place we'd rather be.

More Distractions: Intensifying Our Craving for the "Perfect" Life

In conjunction with the media, our consumer-oriented society has many ways of distracting us with immediate gratification that do not truly add to our peace and well-being. There is always a new product to fulfill us, or some gadget that will ease our discomfort. If we are lonely, we can call or text friends on our cell phones. If we feel restless, we can surf the Web. And, when we are bored, we can always go shopping. Unfortunately, these avenues to happiness are counterproductive; they increase the desire they are supposed to satisfy. The more we have, the more we want, until our superficial pleasures leave us feeling addicted and hung over.

An increasingly-common way our culture encourages us to escape is through overwork. Statistics show that Americans today work 180 more hours per year than they did 30 years ago—which amounts to almost 23 additional work days per year! Life becomes a business we must manage, and our success depends on how much we produce and how well we control our environment. We have become cogs in a wheel that operates on the principle that "time is money," and the value of our lives becomes measured by how productive we are or how much we can purchase, instead of who we are as people.[5]

Women in particular have borne the brunt of this workaholic ethic, since women who are employed outside the house often come home to a "second shift" of housework and childcare. For some of us, working extra hours is necessary to make ends meet. But for others, overworking is part of a broader dysfunctional lifestyle that ignores the problems of the larger world and seeks satisfaction through individual success and material consumption.[6]

In addition, we now live in a technological world where it's quite possible to pass an entire day sitting in front of the computer, working, playing, or just "surfing" an endless sea of virtual information. What's worse, the very technology that can make our life ultra-comfortable and convenient has cut us off from the physical sensations—the smells, tastes, sounds, sights, and touches—through which we encounter the world. Some of us also spend hours in the car every morning and evening just to get to and from work. A woman describes how her sedentary lifestyle and overwork patterns affected her:

> For most of my life, I was naturally thin. In college my room-mates were envious that I could eat anything without gaining weight. But since I've been working as a computer programmer for the past 12 years, putting in 60 hours a week on average, I've gained over 40 pounds. I feel uncomfortable and have a lot less energy. I don't eat more than I used to, but the only exercise I get is going from my bed to my car to my office and back. I like my job, and the pay is great; but, sometimes I feel like I'm living my life from my neck up, and it gets pretty lonely here in my head.

Many of the "distractions" described can be healthy if we do them in moderation and in ways that are socially, environmentally, and personally responsible. But so often we don't. Instead, we turn to the diversions our culture offers to avoid our problems and to fill the spiritual vacuum. We search for "good health" in the form of a fat-free body not because dieting gives us true peace of mind, body, and spirit, but because it directs our attention *away from* more difficult issues. We consume mass media not to sharpen our minds and expand our hearts, but because it's entertaining and provides an easy avenue of escape. We "shop 'til we drop" to make us feel alive again, but we often do so more out of a consumerism habit than necessity. We drive endless hours in gas-guzzling automobiles that disconnect us from our bodies and destroy the environment, not because we are bad people, but because we have adopted our culture's vision of success, which is based on a philosophy of "more-faster-better."[7]

In the end, the same culture that distracts us from our pain also diverts our attention away from the values we hold most dear. This creates a dysfunctional pattern: *When we are not aligned with our deepest values, we find ourselves looking for peace in all the wrong places.* We seek escape instead of presence, which only increases our suffering and fuels our desire for further distractions. Conditioned to distrust our inherent abundance, we become caught in a vicious cycle of working to consume and consuming to relieve the stress of too much work. Our addiction to food and thinness, work, the media, our consumer-oriented lifestyles, cars, phones, and computers, all point to the same underlying fear: we are afraid of being alone with ourselves. We are afraid of our suffering.

Touching Our Suffering: The Way to Healing

Ironically, our resistance to experiencing pain only deepens the hurt. Healing requires us to move closer to our pain, to get to know it, and ultimately to accept it. And so, we must become intimate with our suffering if we wish to grow beyond the false security and comfort of the narrow little world we have constructed in our search for salvation through thinness.

On the surface this sounds a little insane, perhaps even masochistic. Why should we get in touch with our suffering? How could this possibly help us heal? Paradoxically, the answer is that by accepting our pain instead of resisting it—by letting our hearts break open rather than protecting them—we develop the strength we need to handle our difficulties directly.

Your journey beyond The Religion of Thinness starts when you accept the reality that you have become trapped, that you are suffering, and that you no longer want to live this way.

This is a very painful recognition—perhaps one of the hardest you will ever have to make. There is no easy way to do it. But a good place to begin is simply to practice keeping your heart open. Instead of defending yourself from your pain, let it humble you, pierce you, change you. When you don't harden yourself in reaction to feelings of anxiety, depression, hurt, or shame, you develop what Buddhists call *bodhichitta*. This is what Buddhist teacher Pema Chödrön calls the "soft spot" in each of us, the place that is vulnerable and tender. It is the part of us that is capable of feeling love and compassion for ourselves and others. This is the place we need to return to when we feel ourselves shutting down or checking out. We reconnect with this part of ourselves by staying present to our emotional distress and letting our suffering soften us rather than trying to protect ourselves against it.[8]

Just as no one else knows the inside story of your embattled relationship with food and your body, so no one else knows the particular despair that you bury by starving, obsessing, bingeing, and dieting. Your pain may reflect a traumatic experience you suffered as a child, or possibly as a teenager, or even as an adult. Studies indicate, for example, that a disproportionate number of women with eating problems are survivors of sexual abuse.[9] It may be that you suffer internally as a result of constant exposure to unhealthy relationships, meaningless work, or a general sense of angst and depression. Or you may have been badly injured by broader injustices, like sexism, racism, weight or size prejudice, homophobia, economic instability, or ageism, to name just a few.

Whether your pain is rooted in childhood or adult experiences, whether it was inflicted with violence or a more subtle force, you must become aware of the ways it has made you susceptible to The Religion of Thinness. As you do, you can practice peace with your body by keeping your heart open in the midst of your affliction, instead of trying to get back "in control." When you turn and face your pain this way, the true path of peace opens up before you.

A woman who was recovering from years of compulsive eating describes how she practiced staying open:

> For a long time, I was perfectly aware of how I overate to medicate the pain I had accumulated in the course of my life, but I felt powerless to do anything about it. I didn't have a better way to deal with it. Now, with the help of my therapist and daily prayer, I'm learning how to sit still and be quiet. When I start getting that compulsive feeling, I stop whatever I'm doing and find a way to be alone. If I'm home, I go to my bedroom. If I'm at work, I close my office door. Wherever I am, I shut my eyes and ask for help to just be with whatever comes up for me, rather than soothe myself by eating. It may sound corny, but sometimes I even imagine myself holding my pain like a crying baby.

Imagine what would it be like if you could hold your pain like a crying baby, just being present and loving toward yourself, in the midst of your suffering. What if, instead of numbing yourself by starving or bingeing when you feel fear or emptiness, you sit with these feelings, feel their energy, and embrace them with compassion? How would it feel if, instead of trying to control them, you simply let them be—without needing to "figure them out" or "work through" them? The pain itself may not go away (at least not right away), but at least you wouldn't be creating more suffering by feeding your obsession. And, you would be taking a big, courageous step forward in the direction of health and sanity.

This path is open to you right now. You don't need to be any more spiritually advanced or emotionally mature than you already are to experience such healing. You just have to learn how to be mindful of your pain and loving toward yourself. Following is an exercise to help you do that.

Touching Your Suffering: An Exercise in Mindfulness

This exercise[10] is divided into two parts. In Part I, I offer some techniques that will help you use your sensory perception to bring you into the present moment. You will engage your senses to become mindful of your external environment and bring your awareness into your body. This will help you stay grounded when you focus on your internal experiences in the second part of the exercise.

In Part II, I ask you to recall a painful incident from the history of your struggle with food and body image, and to experience the feelings that come up as you remember this event as clearly and completely as possible. You will be asked to "touch," accept, and send loving kindness to the suffering of this one incident, which in turn will broaden your capacity to accept other painful experiences you encounter. This exercise will expand your ability to love and accept even those parts of you that feel unlovable. In this sense it can help lead you to the good health, wholeness, and peace you deserve.

Let's begin.

Part I: Using Your Senses to Return to the Present

- *Watch your breath.* Start by sitting and watching your breath, just as we have done in other exercises throughout this book. Set aside some time to sit quietly in a space where you won't be distracted. Make sure your posture is straight, your shoulders relaxed, and that you are breathing from your belly. Then direct your attention to the air flowing in and out of your body. Just observe this movement for the next few moments.

- *Become mindful of what you hear and smell.* To help you bring your awareness fully into the present moment, focus on your sense of hearing and smell. What noises do you notice as you sit quietly? Do you hear the sound of a washing machine? Your neighbor's lawn mower? Cars driving by? Listen carefully, be curious, and give whatever you hear your full attention. Then turn your attention to any smells in your environment. Is someone in your home cooking dinner? Is the pavement outside wet with rain? Be aware of any odors you detect, pleasant or unpleasant. Do you notice any nuances or subtleties in these scents you didn't notice before?

- ***Become mindful of what you see.*** Once you have experienced your sense of hearing and smell for a while, let go of these sensations and bring your awareness to what you see around you. Sink further into the present moment as you do so. Direct your attention toward an object in the room where you are sitting. Without getting up, look at the object in detail. See it as though you were noticing it for the first time. Look at its colors, textures, contours, and size. Notice where the object ends and the space around it begins. Be mindful of your concentrated state of awareness.

- ***Become mindful of your bodily experience.*** Now close your eyes and bring your attention to your body and the sensations you are having right now. Give it the same kind of undivided attention you gave the objects of your perceptions of smell, hearing, and seeing. What physical sensations are you having in this moment? Can you feel the air move in and out of your lungs and belly? Can you sense your heart beating as it pumps blood to different parts of your body? Bring your attention to these various parts— your toes, feet, legs, hips, stomach, arms, the tips of your fingers, all the way up to your head. Do you experience pleasure or pain in any particular part? Can you sense the life energy that animates your body, as you did in the exercise in Chapter 4?

Part II: Tuning in to Your Pain

- ***Remember a food or body-related incident that caused you pain.*** Staying mindful of your inner experience, turn your attention to a specific food or body-related incident in your life that has caused you pain. It could be the first time someone called you "fat" or a particular night of bingeing and purging. Maybe it's a time when your addiction to food and thinness damaged your relationship with someone you love or prevented you from doing something you really wanted to do. Whatever episode you choose, try to remember it in as much detail as you can. How old were you? Who else was there? Where were you when it happened? What were you wearing? Can you recall any particular sounds or smells?

- *Return to the present moment.* Gently persevere until the incident you are remembering has come fully into your consciousness. As you start to feel the pain of this memory, bring your attention back to your breath and the room you are in. Remember that you are sitting here, now, in the present moment. What happened in the past is in the past. This memory is just a thought in your mind, a mental image. Try to stay grounded in what is true in this moment as you return to your memory and focus again on the details of the experience.

- *Become mindful of your feelings.* As the full picture of this experience forms in your mind, bring your complete awareness to the emotions that come up for you. Try not to label these feelings. When you do, you are actually thinking about them, instead of directly experiencing them. If you start to feel sad or scared, don't focus on the thought "I am sad," or "I am scared." Just notice it as a thought and become present to the feeling itself.

- *Focus on a particular feeling.* If several emotions come up for you, choose one and focus on it (i.e., sadness, fear, anger, shame, etc.). Where is this feeling in your body? Is it in your heart, your stomach, your head? Try to sense how it feels. Is it heavy? Tight? Vulnerable? Empty? If this emotion had a shape, what shape would it be? If it had a color, what color would it be? What kind of energy does this feeling have? Does it hum as though it were alive, or does it feel dull, lethargic, and dim?

- *Stay present to the uncomfortable feeling.* Rather than run from this uncomfortable feeling, see if you can stay present to it as it is. You aren't trying to change it into something it isn't. Nor are you trying to *make* it go away. If that happens, it will happen on its own. For now, try to just sit with the feeling without resisting it *and* without becoming attached to it. Continue being mindful that you are sitting here, in the present, in this room. As you sit here now, see if you can stay with this painful feeling. You aren't promising to do this forever. You aren't justifying whatever happened in the past. You are just experimenting with identifying and being present to your pain, instead of denying or escaping it.

- *Consciously accept your suffering.* Now that you are fully present to your suffering, you have an opportunity to *consciously accept it*—to willingly and intentionally let it be without trying to control it. This feeling is a part of you. It may not be your favorite part. You may wish that the event that sparked this feeling had never happened. You may work to make sure that such an event never occurs again. But the feeling itself is there inside you and is part of who you are right now. You can continue trying to resist it, but so far that approach hasn't brought you much peace. Here is an opportunity to do things differently. I encourage you to take a risk.

- *Remember you are more than your pain.* Although the pain you have become conscious of is a part of you, remember it isn't *all* of you. It's only a fraction of the whole of who you are. It's one feeling from one situation from one part of your history. Is your heart large enough to contain this feeling? And if you reject it, where else will it go? What if your attempt to disown this suffering has been preventing you from feeling whole?

- *Practice compassion towards yourself.* As you consciously accept your pain, see if you can send it loving kindness. This dark, difficult part of you is still worth loving. More than anything, it needs your compassion. Think of it as a rebellious child who, beneath her tough veneer, needs nothing more than to feel accepted for who she is. See if you can embrace the soft spot you've been guarding with food and thinness. Once you have uncovered and touched it, you can take better care of it. Carry it with you as you would a child. Give it the compassion it needs to heal, and become the Great Mother that you are.

- *Extend your compassion to others who suffer.* Once you have experienced compassion towards yourself, you are ready to take the final step in this exercise and share it with others. Call to mind some of the people you know who are suffering. These can be friends, family members, neighbors, or people you have never met. With your heart wide open, send them as much compassion as you can, and make a wish that they may be at peace. As you do this, realize that your private pain is part of a much larger river of human hurt. This does not invalidate or diminish the personal suffering *you* have experienced, but it places it in a broader perspective, alongside the billions of other people who have experienced loss, disappointment, depression, fear, and all those feelings that make us want to run and hide. Ultimately, offering compassion to others who are hurting, both people you know and people you don't, is a profoundly inclusive healing gesture.

You can use this exercise to touch other painful experiences in your life and to accept difficulties as they arise. In fact, the exercise will be more useful if you use it regularly and repeatedly rather than trying it once and forgetting about it. This exercise isn't intended (nor can it work) as a cure-all. It won't end your disordered eating overnight. But little-by-little it can help you learn to be increasingly loving and compassionate toward yourself. In so doing, it can slowly but surely lead you to that peaceful place inside, the place where you can accept and love yourself exactly as you are—the yin and the yang, good and bad, beautiful and ugly—inclusive of both angels and demons.

Befriending Our Demons: Reconciling Ourselves with Desire

In fact, in some traditional religions, human appetites and urges are sometimes represented as *demons:* invisible forces that distract or corrupt spiritual seekers by manipulating their basic desires and pleasures. Whether they are personified as agents of evil or represented as inner cravings, stories of demons point to the human tendency to search for salvation in the wrong places. Our desire for satisfying relationships gets clouded by the "demons" of loneliness or lust. Our longing for a larger sense of purpose gets caught up in a race for power and prestige. Our need for resources to support our well-being becomes haunted by a greedy fear that we can never get enough. And our hunger for food gets seduced by the pleasure of overeating or the pride of excessive abstaining.

While demons typically represent negative influences, their function is not entirely evil. In many religious myths and legends, they are depicted as fallen gods or angels, and encounters with them can fortify the commitment of spiritual seekers. Jesus' struggle in the wilderness, where the Devil tempts him with food, power, and authority, only strengthens his resolve to fulfill his true calling (Matthew 4:1–11; Luke 4:1–13). The story of the Buddha reveals a similar pattern when, on the verge of enlightenment, he is attacked by the Lord of Desire (in the form of a voluptuous woman) and the Lord of Death (in the form of hurricanes, torrential rains, and showers of flaming rocks). As legend has it, the Buddha had developed his practice of non-attachment so well that the instruments of these demonic assaults turned into flower petals as they entered the field of his concentration.

These examples underscore the fundamental ambiguity of the

desires that demons represent: their destructive as well as their creative potential. There is little question that our cravings can be harmful; they can propel shortsighted thinking and behaviors that injure ourselves and others. But they can also be life-giving; they can inspire insights and actions that enhance our own health and the well-being of others. The powerful energy of our yearnings can lead to selfishness, or it can call us beyond ourselves. We can allow our demons to lead us into temptation, or we can use them to deliver us from "evil."

As we try to recover from our disordered relationship with food and our bodies, many of us may fall into the trap of believing that our "eating disorder" is something we must "overcome." It begins to look like a problem that must be solved if we are going to be free and finally find peace, like a demon that must be exorcised if we are ever to achieve the dream of good health.

It is true that we need to make a conscious choice to let go of our attachment to The Religion of Thinness if we wish to be free of its power. We must learn to see through the cultural mechanisms that support it, identify the spiritual needs that draw us to it, and examine how these have influenced our attitudes toward our bodies and the food we do or do not eat. We need to be persistent in our efforts to remain mindful, practice peace with our bodies, critique the messages we consume, and find alternative ways of meeting our spiritual hungers so that we are less inclined to engage in thought patterns and behaviors that are ultimately self-defeating.

However, a problem arises when we start holding on too tightly to the idea that our disordered relationship with food and our bodies is something that needs to be excised once and for all: we start a new war with ourselves. Our battle with weight and eating turns into a war against the disorder itself, and we perpetuate the same mentality that got us into trouble in the first place—we desperately want to eradicate that part of us that feels shameful, ugly, dark, painful, and needy. Just as The Religion of Thinness taught us to believe that we should be able to subdue our appetites and bodies, so now, as we begin the journey of recovery, we may be tempted to think we should be able to "conquer" our eating and body image problems.

When this happens, every time we slip and "fall off the wagon," every time we binge, purge, starve, or monitor our calories, we are prone to judge ourselves—and we usually judge pretty harshly. We badger ourselves with questions like: "Why can't I stop these stupid behaviors?" "Why can't I eat like a normal person?" And we often conclude that we're just "too weak," "too sick in the head," or "too emotionally (or spiritually) immature" to be able to heal.

And yet, you won't find peace "once you are free from your food problems" anymore than you will find peace "once you are thin." You can only experience peace *now*. That means you are going to have to find a way to bring your body image issues and disordered eating *along with you* on this journey of healing.

The reality is that this *is* a journey with lots of lessons. You'll be cleaning up the kitchen after dinner one night and suddenly realize that you've been adding up the calories you just consumed, at which point you may stop and think, "There I go again." Or you'll realize that the first thing you thought about when your sister told you she was getting married is how you would look in a bridesmaid dress, but you refuse to buy into the female ritual of losing weight before a wedding. Or maybe you'll get depressed because things aren't working out right in a relationship, and you'll find yourself looking for comfort in ice cream, but will stop yourself after just a few bites. When these kinds of ocurrences happen, you have a choice: you can beat yourself up for not being more "perfect," or you can reflect on what happened, learn from it, let it go, and start anew by practicing loving kindness toward yourself. You can condemn and try to punish or suppress your "demon," or you can befriend it by accepting it for what it is: a struggle you are having at this point in your life.

On the surface, accepting this struggle may sound like a contradiction to everything I have been talking about in this book. But paradoxically, it is the very *core* of what I am talking about. Befriending this demon—your eating problem—is perhaps one of the biggest steps you can take on your road to healing.

Befriending your demon doesn't mean engaging in your habitual self-destructive patterns whenever the desire hits you. It means becoming mindful of your feelings and urges as they arise without trying to make them go away, sending loving kindness toward them and towards the parts of your spirit that feel most damaged, accepting yourself as you are, practicing peace with your body, and realizing you are already a whole human being, in this moment, warts and all.

Acceptance is the road to holistic good health. This includes accepting how you sometimes abuse food and your body. Whether this "demon" is a relatively new intruder in your life, or whether you've lived with it for decades, it's a part of who you are. Although it has caused you so much pain, it has also brought you to *this point*—one where you are ready for change.

In this way, accepting your struggle as *essential* for your health and healing allows you to turn your recovery "failures" into opportunities for growth. Can you notice what the energy of acceptance feels like? It is open, trusting, willing, soft, and yet somehow also enduringly strong. This energy of acceptance converts an "enemy" into a friend. It enables you to see your relapses and frustrations as chances to practice peace with your body once again. Accepting your struggle for what it is enables you to think of your setbacks as perfect occasions for training yourself to practice compassion rather than judgment, to stay present instead of trying to escape, to persevere with patience when you'd rather give up.

The path of nonresistance I'm describing here presents an alternative to the frustrating road you have traveled for far too long. There's no guarantee where this path will lead. Your disordered relationship with food and your body may completely resolve one day, or it may not. But you can begin to plant seeds of peace in its very ground right now in this moment. Your suffering has created fertile soil in which these seeds can grow, if you give them the loving care they need.

It's hard to believe that the very demons that have caused you so much suffering and self-destruction can become creative and life-giving forces in your life. But take a minute to think about it: where did your eating behaviors come from in the first place? From a desire to be a better person, from the longing to feel happy and free, from your yearning to experience the peace and good health of salvation. If these demons could eventually lead you to a path for truly achieving these things, then couldn't they indeed become guiding angels?

Unfortunately, when we think of our drive to starve, binge, purge, or diet as bad or sinful, and fight our urges, we repress not just the desire we think is destructive, but also the underlying hunger that is creative and fertile. In so doing, we cut ourselves off from an important source of empowerment and motivation for healing: our passion.

Turning Our Demons into Angels: Embracing Our Passion

Women who engage in disordered eating or body refinement often do so because they are looking for an outlet for their passion—a meaningful way to engage the dynamic life force within them.

Passion is an interesting word. In the original Latin it meant "suffering." For example, the "passion of Christ," refers to his suffering. In fact, the first definition for "passion" in *Merriam-Webster's Collegiate Dictionary (11th Edition)* is "the sufferings of Christ between the night of the Last Supper and his death." Nowadays, the term often connotes an "intense, driving, overmastering feeling or conviction." And, of course, sometimes the word is used interchangeably with sexual desire.

When I say that women engage in eating disorders because they are looking for a meaningful outlet for their passion, I use the word to include both suffering and desire, because I don't think they can be separated. The things we feel strongest about are also the things that have the most power to make us suffer. The people we love the most can cause us the worst pain. The causes we care about deeply are the ones that can break our hearts when they don't work out as we had hoped. This intense mixture of suffering and desire has a kind of embodied, sensual, earthy quality to it, which is perhaps why it is often associated with sexuality. We experience passion not just in our heads, but throughout our body, with our whole being, and its power can feel invigorating or seductive, uplifting or scary, angelic or demonic. Our passion has the power to hurt us and to heal us. It is our life force. If life is suffering, then life is passion.

There are many reasons you may have been driven to pour your passion into the pursuit of thinness. We've explored some in this book. We've seen how our society makes it seem like a worthy cause, and how the promises The Religion of Thinness offers are quite attractive and appeal to our spiritual hungers. But we've also seen how empty and damaging these promises are, and how we need alternative ways to create meaning in our lives and to reconnect with the life-force within us.

While much has been written about the need for emotional healing in the process of recovery from disordered eating, less attention is given to integrating the passions masked by these problems and finding healthier outlets for them. These needs are interrelated. We cannot begin to explore our deepest desires with our inner wounds still fresh and bleeding. But healing is virtually impossible without some bigger motivation to recover. At some point, we have to discover those parts of ourselves that inspire us to thrive on our journey. To experience the wholeness we misguidedly seek in the form of a perfect body, we must recognize and address the longings and needs that get buried in our preoccupation with food. We must identify where our true passions lie. We must reconnect with our ultimate purpose.

Can you remember something you felt passionate about before you became absorbed in the world of weight-loss and calories? What desires and goals did you have? What causes did you care about? To what were you devoted? What energized your mind, body, and spirit? What made you feel truly alive? If, like so many other women, your preoccupation with food and thinness has caused you to lose touch with your deepest yearnings, your recovery presents an opportunity to rediscover them.

Strengthening Our Connection to the Truths We Hold Sacred

When our attention is focused on weight and thinness, our lives do not reflect the deepest values of our hearts. But by reconnecting to our physical body and learning to have faith in the life force that sustains us, we offer ourselves an opportunity to reconnect to that which we most cherish. As authors Lynn Ginsburg and Mary Taylor write, "When we've lost a spiritual connection in our lives, we may eat and eat in an attempt to fill our inner void. But satisfaction comes only when we're able to rediscover our connection to whatever holds deepest meaning for us."[11]

Remembering what really matters in life is something humans have been struggling with for ages. Traditional religions recognize this difficulty. In Islam, the tendency to forget what is most important is considered the tragedy of the human condition. This is why devout Muslims pray five times a day. Prayer strengthens a person's connection to God and therefore reconnects Muslims with what is most essential to them. In the words of the Prophet Muhammad, "Remembering God is the cure for the heart."[12]

Throughout the day, especially when we find ourselves preoccupied by food and thinness, we can practice peace with our bodies by revisiting a few basic questions:

- What do I hold sacred?
- What is it that truly gives my life meaning?
- What is the ultimate purpose of my life?
- Is what I am choosing or doing in alignment with my core values?

Questions like these slow us down and help us remember what we already know to be true, namely, that our health, peace, and fulfillment do not depend on having a "perfect" body, and that we do not have to be "perfect" people to experience the peace of heaven around and within us.

There are a number of ways we can keep these questions at the center of our lives, including any of the mindfulness practices in this book. Perhaps the most common is the simple practice of prayer.

Using Prayer to Focus on Your Ultimate Purpose

Prayer means many different things to different people. But whatever form it takes, prayer is essentially a means for staying in touch with the questions and truths that give our lives meaning. It helps us to stay present to what really matters, and this fortifies our spirits when our thoughts turn to The Religion of Thinness.

Some of us have traditional prayers. "When I find myself feeling anxious about food or whatever else is giving me a hard time in life, I start singing the prayer of St. Francis," a recovering bulimic woman explains:

> The words of that prayer—"Make me a channel of your peace; where there is hatred let me bring Your love; where there is injury Your pardon, Lord; and where there's doubt true faith in You"—put me back in a frame of mind that is peaceful. From there, I know I can make healthy decisions.

In addition to (or instead of) traditional prayers, some of us may turn to the embodied forms of prayer discussed in Chapter 4 of this book (i.e., mindfully connecting with the power of life in our bodies, practicing yoga, engaging in social activism). Or, we may draw on the sacred symbols we've discovered in the course of our recovery. A Catholic woman who was healing from years of body-hatred developed the practice of silently reciting her own version of the "Hail Mary" before eating breakfast each morning:

> Hail Mary, full of grace, may your wisdom be with me.
> Blessed are you, as are all women, and
> Blessed is the fruit of our hearts, our minds, and our bodies.
> Holy Mary, mother of God,
> Pray for me, my children, and all beings,
> Now and at the hour of our death. Amen.

Whatever formulas, techniques, and symbols we use, praying is a way to strengthen our connection with the truths we hold sacred, and this gives us the courage and trust we need to accept our lives—and our bodies—as they are. A woman who spent years loathing her body and restricting her eating explains how the practice of daily prayer helped her accept her life and see it from a broader perspective:

> For a long time, I wasn't comfortable praying because my only experience with prayer was what I learned at church and that really didn't do anything for me. But in the course of my recovery, I've learned to pray in my own way. It's not about bargaining with God or promising to be "good" so I'll get rewarded. Instead, I just ask for help in remembering what my life's really about—like being a kind and loving person, trying to do my part to help out in this messed-up world, and feeling at peace with myself no matter what happens. Taking time out of every day to center myself in these core values gives me strength when I feel myself sliding back into negative self-talk or other unhealthy habits.

Another form of prayer that some women use to counteract such negative self-talk is the repetition of a mantra, a word or phrase which, when repeated, returns our awareness to the peace that is already in us. While mantras are often associated with eastern traditions, like the Sanskrit *"om,"* every religion has its own. Muslims repeat the name of God. Jews say "Shema Yisrael," ("Hear, Israel") or simply "Shalom" ("peace," "wholeness," "well-being"). "Come Lord Jesus" is a mantra for Christians. One of the most ancient and basic mantras in India, *Râma,* comes from the Sanskrit root *ram,* "to rejoice," signifying the source of peace and joy.[13] Reciting a mantra is a unique way of praying because the sound of the truth repeated resonates throughout the entire person, unifying body, mind, and spirit. The Hindu yogi Yogananda suggests that such verbal affirmations stimulate the healing energy in our bodies, increasing our overall sense of well-being. Patient, persistent, and attentive repetition of our spiritual truths strengthens our connection to our inner wisdom.[14]

In the Sufi Muslim tradition, the practice of "remembrance," in which the name of God is repeated, is a technique for opening the heart and connecting believers to the power of life both beyond and within them. The Whirling Dervishes, who practice spinning their bodies continuously to enter into a meditative state, are a branch of this tradition. As they spin, the dervishes strive to unify their breath and movement with the sound of the name of the one who sustains them.[15] Through their physical turning, the gravity of the world is loosened, along with the pull of its anxieties and empty pleasures. Dervishes are said to cross the threshold between matter and spirit, uniting them with the power of the God. The founder of the Whirling Dervishes, a 13th-century Sufi named Rumi, saw life as a love affair between the human soul and the divine. When our attention is fully concentrated on God, the creative power of the universe acts through us.

Some of us may find it helpful to create personal mantras specifically designed to promote a sense of harmony between our bodies, minds, and spirits. Quietly repeating words like "acceptance," "strength," "truth," or "courage" when we feel ourselves tightening with fear can return us to the present moment. This is another practice we can do anytime, anywhere: sitting still on a meditation cushion, kneeling quietly in a church, peeling carrots in front of the sink, or driving the kids to school. When we find ourselves resorting to our old, self-critical habits, we can use our mantra to affirm what we know to be true. If we practice repeatedly, it may eventually become as second nature to us as the lies about thinness we once held dear.

Affirmations are also an effective way to reinforce positive self-talk. We can start our day saying them aloud in front of a mirror, being fully present to the words as we speak. Or we can say them silently after (or before) meditating or praying. "I will live free from fear today," "I am strong, intelligent, caring, and beautiful," "I am capable of handling whatever happens to me today," "I have something positive to contribute to the world," are just a few examples. You may feel disingenuous saying them at first. But if practiced repeatedly, the meaning of affirmations like these will sink in and take root deep in your psyche.

Each of us must find our own way of reconnecting with our ultimate purpose. The important thing is that we develop ways to remain mindful of the truths that open our hearts and nourish our spirits as we struggle against the currents of our old habit of searching for salvation through thinness.

This may sound like a serious undertaking. But it doesn't have to be somber. In fact, one of the most powerful ways to reconnect with and learn to trust the abundance of life is to rediscover your capacity for play.

Rediscovering Your Capacity for Play: Enjoying Your Path of Recovery

Through our relentless dedication to thinness, many of us have forgotten what it's like to have fun. It's hard to be spontaneous when we're feeling shameful, and our rigid approach to our appetites and desires often makes us resentful. Likewise, our path to recovery can be a lot of work. We get bogged down in trying to change old patterns and forget that we can enjoy our lives in the process. Learning to live more fully *in* your body is a way of bringing more joy to your life. It is also one of the most effective ways to stay grounded in your sacred values, to resist the influence of The Religion of Thinness, and to heal the damage it has caused you.

Since your eating disorder is not just in your head, neither will your healing be. You can't *think* your way out of this problem. You have to find healthy alternatives to your obsessive behaviors—creative endeavors that fully engage your mind, body, and spirit; activities in which you become so involved that nothing else seems to matter. You need life-giving outlets for your passions, especially ones that create the experience of "flow"[16] and allow you to let go of control without losing yourself. These "in the zone" experiences can be tremendously healing because they teach us how to be *in* our bodies and to trust the abundance of our lives.

Loosening our grip on the steering wheel for a while and forgetting about all our destinations means being present to our lives as they are *right now*—not someday when we lose enough weight. When we do this, we become like children engrossed in play: not concerned about the past or the future; not worried about what others think; not preoccupied with the "flaws" of our legs, stomach, or hips; not thinking about anything other than what we are doing. We just are where we are, doing what we're doing, immersed in life and fully present in our bodies. This kind of mindful attention is not only very relaxing but also a lot of fun! Being completely in our bodies frees us to be in the here and now, without some big agenda of how things are supposed to be, without regret about what could have been, and without waiting to be "thin enough." This is not just the key to enjoying our bodies; it is also the secret to enjoying our lives.

To create these kinds of experiences we must find activities that relax us and that increase our capacity for play. How can you do this? Try asking yourself some simple questions: What do I really enjoy doing? What activities give me both peace and pleasure and leave me feeling replenished and whole? These questions may lead you to rediscover the pleasurable endeavors you let fall by the wayside as your focus on food and thinness became more consuming. Or they might inspire you to find wholly new ways to have fun inside your body. You might try making a list of things you once loved to do and no longer engage in, or things you've always wanted to try but have never gotten around to. Here are just a few examples to get you started:

- Gardening
- Horseback or bike riding
- Hiking
- Needlepoint, sewing, or other crafts
- Practicing martial arts
- Yoga
- Sports
- Playing a musical instrument
- Cooking cuisine from other cultures
- Dancing
- Getting a massage or taking a spa bath
- Drawing or painting

Activities like these replenish us by giving us a break from our ordinary strivings and worries. When our bodies and spirits are centered in activities that capture our undivided attention, our minds are free to be creative. Liberated from the scheming, controlling, inflexible, futuristic mentality of The Salvation of Thinness, we can experience the joy of *now.*

Both returning to activities we know we love and exploring unfamiliar new ones can enhance our lives. A recovering anorexic woman, for example, rediscovered her love of sports:

> I was a pretty good athlete before I gave my life over to calories and thinness. Basketball was my favorite sport. Something about the feel of the ball bouncing back-and-forth between my hand and the floor put my mind at ease. After practices, and especially after games, I always had this feeling of my mind being washed clean. Now, as part of my recovery, I've rounded up a group of women who used to play and we shoot hoops in the park a few times a week. We're not as young or as quick as we used to be, but it's a lot of fun and it helps me keep a sense of humor.

There are many things we can do to close the gaps between our minds, bodies, and spirits. The activities you choose are not as important as the attention you bring to them. Walking around the neighborhood can be as invigorating as climbing a mountain if you are mindful of what you are doing. A young woman recovering from anorexia and bulimia describes how music became a means for experiencing the peace and pleasure of being in her body:

> I used to rely on starving and bingeing as a way to soothe my anxiety and give myself that "everything's-going-to-be-okay" feeling. But as I'm learning more balanced ways of eating, music has become a new source of comfort. I especially like listening to jazz. Improvisation is something I need to work on—not in music but in my life. I also like music that's easy to sing with. When I sing along with my favorite songs, something inside of me shifts. Singing lightens my mood and my body.

Engaging in activities that allow us to get "in the zone" is not a way to escape our insecurities and pain; it is how we learn to give our rational, calculating selves a break and open up to something bigger. This process of opening teaches us to trust in something other than our own abilities to control our bodies, something that empowers us with the deep-seated awareness that we already have everything we need to be peaceful and whole.

This trust is not the same as blind faith. It isn't based on denying our problems, and it doesn't put our critical consciousness to sleep. On the contrary, letting go of our need to be in control frees us to be present to reality as it is—problems and all—rather than how we wish it would be. By practicing loving kindness and being in our bodies, rather than trying to conquer or escape them, we can begin to have faith that the power of life that transcends and flows through us will provide the strength we need to handle whatever comes our way. As we learn to trust this gracious, empowering presence—even and especially when we feel most stuck and afraid—we open ourselves to the peace of mind, body, and spirit that we truly crave.

Reasons to Hope

Although there is no magical cure for our eating and body image problems, there are good reasons to hope that we can enjoy the "good health" and peace of salvation. Hope is essential for healing. We have to believe that we *can* learn to enjoy life in our bodies and in this world. But for hope to be something other than wishful thinking, it needs to be rooted in practice.

As I have explained throughout this book, we practice peace in a multitude of ways by:

- sharing our critical insights with others and cultivating relationships with like-minded people who support our commitment to recovery and spiritual growth

- paying attention to our bodies' signals and eating and exercising in ways that are nourishing

- choosing new role models and images to guide our self-discovery and definition

- creating alternative rituals that give us stability and move us through the changes around and within us

- becoming more accountable to ourselves and others through our everyday thoughts and choices

- "stepping off the capitalist treadmill," as Eve Ensler put it,[17] and challenging a consumer-oriented culture that encourages us to go to war with our bodies

- slowing down and using our breath to help us stay present to the feelings that scare us

- strengthening our connection to the truths we hold sacred

- engaging in activities that allow us to let go without losing ourselves

Through these and other yet-to-be-created practices, we transform not just our relationship to food and our bodies, but also the meaning of our lives: our sense of who we are and what we have to contribute to the world.

We can also be hopeful because our personal transformation is part of a larger cultural revolution that is already underway. I have shared what I know about some of the movements and organizations dedicated to creating a world in which all bodies can flourish. In addition to these, there are countless individual women who are waking up and seeing through the lies that keep The Religion of Thinness in business. The findings of a 2004 global study entitled "The Real Truth About Beauty" make this trend evident. Thirty-two-hundred women from around the world, ages 18-64, participated in this study, which was commissioned by Dove. The vast majority felt that manufactured, mass-produced images of female beauty were limiting and inauthentic. Seventy-five percent of them said they'd like to see considerably more diversity in terms of size, shape, color, and age in media images of women. And two-thirds of them strongly agreed that a woman's beauty is defined more by her character—her dignity, happiness, kindness, wisdom, love, integrity, and self-realization—than by her physical appearance.[16]

As this study suggests, those of us who are fed up with our culture's narrow ideal are not alone in our journey. Even as the Religion of Thinness continues to circulate beliefs, images, rituals, and rules that entice us to worship the fat-free form, a growing number of us are deciding to change our minds instead of our bodies, to reshape society instead of our figures. Beautiful, brave, intelligent women everywhere are choosing to devote their energies to creating a world in which all bodies are loved and cared for. Soccer moms and college students, girls and grandmothers, corporate executives and administrative assistants, doctors, lawyers, artists, salesclerks, teachers, nurses, businesswomen and homemakers, women from small towns and big cities across the U.S. and around the globe are waking up and realizing that beneath our drive for thinness lies a deeper hunger for a life that is meaningful and whole.

You can be part of this revolution. In fact, through your everyday thoughts, choices, and interactions, you can help it spread. You can talk with all the people who matter in your life about *your* decision to start loving your body rather than constantly berating or fighting it. Choosing to participate in this personal-social transformation can generate the confidence and courage you'll need to persist in your efforts to transform your suffering and discover the larger purpose of your life.

It's never too late to learn to love your body. You can start right now by taking a deep, slow breath and feeling the energy moving within. You can decide that for today, or even for the next hour, you're going to treat your body with loving-kindness. If thoughts about food and thinness start to occupy your mind, you can notice them, smile as you take another deep breath, and then find ways to nurture yourself. Listen to music, go for a walk, say a prayer, or do whatever else you can to center yourself and calm your spirit. And when the day or hour is up, you can choose to renew your decision. You don't have to worry about the future because the only time you can truly practice peace with your body is right now, in this very moment.

If you want to move beyond The Religion of Thinness, then, to paraphrase the wisdom of Mahatma Gandhi, *you must become the change you hope to see in yourself and in society.* If, in addition to your own healing, you want your daughters and granddaughters and people of all generations, genders, colors, shapes, and sizes to be able to live peacefully in their bodies, then you must continue treating *yours* with respect and kindness. As you do, you embody and radiate the values— love, compassion, integrity, and courage—that you want to experience not only in your own life, but also in the world.

ENDNOTES

INTRODUCTION

[1] In its 393-page study entitled "The U.S. Weight Loss & Diet Control Market (9th edition), Marketdata Enterprises, Inc., reports that Americans spent $58 billion trying to lose weight in 2007, and projects a 6% annual growth rate for this market, which puts the number at $68.7 billion by 2010. See www.prwebdirect.com/releases/2007/4/prweb520127.php). See also Stephanie Saul, "Sales Are Strong for Glaxo's Weight-Loss Product," *New York Times*, (Oct. 24, 2007): 2; Sandra O'Loughlin, "Marketers of the Next Generation," *Brandweek* 48:16 (April 2007): 21–26; and Marcia Mogelonsky and Shannon Dortch, "Diets and Deals," *American Demographics* 18:10 (1996): 28. For other statistics related to the diet industry, see Laura Fraser, *Losing It: America's Obsession with Weight and the Industry that Feeds On It* (New York: Dutton, 1997). On the sale of diet books and the Bible, see Roberta Pollack Seid, *Never Too Thin: Why Women Are at War with Their Bodies* (New York: Prentice Hall, 1989), 4, 21. For more on the popularity of diet books, see Better Nutrition Staff, "New Year, New You, New Diet?" *Better Nutrition* 68:1 (January 2006): 56–59; Bob Minzeheimer, "Best-Selling Books List Turns 15 Years of Pages of Top Sellers," *USA Today* (Oct. 30, 2008); and Marketdata Enterprises, "The U.S. Weight Loss & Diet Control Market," (10th Edition, February 2009).

[2] For statistics on anorexia and bulimia, see W. Cromie, "One in Five Female Undergraduates Has Eating Problem," *Harvard University Gazette* 88 (May 7, 1993): 3, 10; K.A. Halmi et al., "Binge Eating and Vomiting: A Survey of A College Population," *Psychological Medicine* 11 (1981): 697–706; S. Nevo, "Bulimic Symptoms: Prevalence and Ethnic Differences among College Women," *International Journal of Eating Disorders* 4 (1985): 151–68.

[3] M.G. Thompson and D.M. Schwartz, "Life Adjustment of Women with Anorexia Nervosa and Anorexic-like Behavior," *International Journal of Eating Disorders* 1 (1982): 47–60; see also S. Nevo, "Bulimic Symptoms," 151–68.

[4] Cristine I. Celio, et al., "Use of Diet Pills and Other Diet Aids in a College Population with High Weight and Shape Concerns," *International Journal of Eating Disorders* 39:6 (2006): 492–497.

[5] Such episodes are cited in articles by Courtney Rubin, "When Only a First Name Is Used" *Washingtonian* (May 2000): p. 58 and Erin Kennedy, "Miss California Talks to Students About Eating Disorders," *Fresno Bee* (November 20, 2004): B1. See also "Speaking Out on Bulimia Book Triggered Flood of Letters by Readers with Eating Disorders," *San Antonio Express-News* (February 1, 1993): 19A; and Barbara DiObilda, "Author Finally Beats Bulimia, Tosses Out the Bathroom Scale," *Houston Chronicle* (Jan 3, 1993): 14.

[6] The greater prevalence of binge eating disorder (BED) is discussed in Diann M. Ackard, et al., "Prevalence and Utility of DSM-IV Eating Disorder Diagnostic Criteria among Youth," *International Journal of Eating Disorders* 40 (2007): 409–417; it is additionally reported in Nicholas Bakalar's article "Survey Puts New Focus on Binge Eating as a Diagnosis," *New York Times* (February 13, 2007); see also James Hudson, et al., "The Prevalence and Correlates of Eating Disorders in the National Comorbidity Survey Replication," *Biological Psychiatry* 61:3 (February 2007): 348–358.

[7] See Halmi et al., "Binge Eating and Vomiting," 683–691; R. C. Hawkins and P. F. Clement, "Development and Construct Validation of a Self-Report Measure of Binge Eating Tendencies," *Addictive Behaviors* 5(1980): 219–226.

[8] P. F. Sullivan, "Mortality in Anorexia Nervosa," 152:7 *American Journal of Psychiatry* (1995): 1073–1074. See also Kathryne L. Westin's "Testimony Before the Subcommittee on Health of the House Committee on Ways and Means," March 27, 2007, accessible at: http://waysandmeans.house.gov/hearings. asp?formmode=view&id=5745. Kitty Westin founded the Anna Westin Eating Disorders Coalition for Research, Policy, and Action, as well as the Anna Westin Foundation, a non-profit dedicated to the prevention and treatment of eating disorders.

[9] These statistics are cited by Jean Kilbourne in *Deadly Persuasion: Why Women and Girls Must Fight the Addictive Power of Advertising* (New York: The Free Press, 1999), 125, 134. According to a *Psychology Today* survey, 62 percent of young women between the ages of 13 and 19 are dissatisfied with their weight. See David Garner, "The Body image Survey Results," *Psychology Today* 30:1 (1997): 30

[10] The percentage for fourth-grade girls is based on a study of 10-year-olds in the Chicago and San Francisco areas. This study is cited by Joan Jacobs Brumberg in *Fasting Girls: The History of Anorexia Nervosa* (New York, 1988), 32. The percentage for women in their mid-50s appears in L. McLaren and D. Kuh, "Body Dissatisfaction in Midlife Women," *Journal of Women and Aging* 16 (2004): 35–55. See also Lynn Brandsma, "Eating Disorders Across the Life Span," *Journal of Women and Aging* 19:1/2 (2007): 155–172

[11] Studies discussing the prevalence of eating problems among women of color include: L. C. Palmer, "Crossing the Color Line: Emerging Realities about Eating Disorders and Treatment with Women of Color," *Journal of Feminist Family Therapy* 19:4 (2007): 21–41; "Eating Disorders in White and Black Women," *Eating Disorders Review* 15:3 (May/June 2004): 5; Ruth Striegel-Moore, et al., "Eating Disorder in White and Black Women," *American Journal of Psychiatry* 160:7 (July 2003): 1326; F. Cachelin, E. Barzegarnazari, and R. H. Striegel-Moore, "Disordered Eating, Acculturation, and Treatment-Seeking in a Community Sample of Hispanic, Asian, Black, and White Women," *Psychology of Women Quarterly* 24 (2000): 244–253; R. H. Striegel-Moore, et al., "Drive for Thinness in Black and White Preadolescent Girls, *International Journal of Eating Disorders* 18:1 (1994): 59–69; D. Wilfley, et al., "Eating Disturbances and Body Image: A Comparison of a Community Sample of Adult Black and White Women," *International Journal of Eating Disorders* 20:4 (1995): 367–377; M. N. Miller and A. J. Pumariega, "Culture and Eating Disorders: A Historical and Cross-Cultural Review," *Psychiatry* 64:2 (2001): 93–110; L. W. Rosen et al., "Prevalence of Pathogenic Weight-Control Behaviors among Native American Women and Girls," *International Journal of Eating Disorders* 7 (1988): 807–11; L. Emmons, "Dieting and Purging Behavior in Black and White High School Students," *Journal of the American Diet Association* 92 (1992): 306–12; L. K. G. Hsu, "Are Eating Disorders Becoming More Common in Blacks?" *International Journal of Eating Disorders* 6 (1987): 113–124; T. J. Silber "Anorexia Nervosa in Blacks and Hispanics," *International Journal of Eating Disorders* 5 (1986): 121–128; Maria Root, "Disordered Eating in Women of Color," *Sex Roles* 22 (1990): 525–536; J. E. Smith and J. Krejci, "Minorities Join the Majority: Eating Disturbances among Hispanic and Native American Youth," *International Journal of Eating Disorders* 10 (1991): 179–186; and L. Osvold and G. Sodowsky, "Eating Disorders of White American, Racial and Ethnic Minority American, and International Women," *Journal of Multicultural Counseling and Development* 21 (1993): 143–154. For a qualitative study of eating problems among women who are ethnically and racially diverse, see Becky Thompson, *A Hunger So Wide and So Deep: American Women Speak Out on Eating Problems* (Minneapolis: University of Minnesota Press, 1994). For issues relating to men's growing dissatisfaction with their bodies, see Arnold Andersen, Leigh Cohn, and Thomas Holbrook's *Making Weight: Men's Conflicts with Food, Weight, Shape and Appearance* (Carlsbad, CA: Gürze, 2000).

[12] Laura Fraser discusses the debates among "obesity researchers" and challenges the conventional wisdom that being overweight is automatically unhealthy in *Losing It!: False Hopes and Fat Promises in the Diet Industry* (New York: Dutton, 1997), 212–235. In his review of 13 studies on obesity and mortality, Ancel Keys concludes that risk of early death increases only when persons are extremely obese or underweight and that weight had no significant impact on the health of the women (80 percent) between these extremes. A. Keys, "Overweight, Obesity, Coronary Heart Disease, and Mortality," *Nutrition Review* 38 (1980): 297–307. Other research shows that obesity is genetically determined rather than consciously chosen. See A. J. Stunkard

et al., "An Adoption Study of Human Obesity," *New England Journal of Medicine* 214 (1986): 193–98. More recently, researchers have discovered what they call the "Obesity Paradox": overweight and obese patients with chronic diseases have better outcomes than their lean counterparts. See Jeptha P. Curtis, et al., "The Obesity Paradox: Body Mass Index and Outcomes in Patients with Heart Failure," *Archives of Internal Medicine* 165:1 (2005): 55–61; and Science Daily, "'Obesity Paradox' Evidence: Obese Patients Fare Better than Lean Patients when Hospitalized for Acute Heart Failure," *Science News* (Jan. 9, 2007), accessed at: www.sciencedaily.com/releases/2007/01/070108145742.htm.

[13] Paul Campos, Abigail Saguy, Paul Oliver, and Glen Gaesser, "The Epidemiology of Overweight and Obesity: Public Health Crisis or Moral Panic?" *International Journal of Epidemiology* 35:1 (2006):55–60; and Abigail Saguy and Kevin Riley, "Weighing Both Sides: Morality, Mortality, and Framing Contests over Obesity," *Journal of Health, Politics, Policy, and Law* 30:5 (2005): 869–921

[14] I say that the authority of organized religion has "in some ways declined" because the trend is not straightforward or simple. Although traditional religious beliefs and institutions are no longer the primary or sole source of authority for many people in the United States and Western Europe, a growing number of people around the world, particularly in the Southern Hemisphere, are turning to organized religions to help them make sense of their life experiences. Even in the United States, the decline of religious devotion among some segments of the population has been accompanied by the rise of fundamentalism and evangelical fervor among others during the past several decades. A good source for some of these trends is Phil Jenkins, *The Next Christendom: The Coming of Global Christianity* (New York: Oxford University Press, 2002).

1

CHANGING THE PARADIGM
From "The Religion of Thinness" to Practicing Peace with Our Bodies

[1] *Marya Hornbacher, Wasted: A Memoir of Anorexia and Bulimia (New York: Harper-Flamingo, 1998).*

[2] www.insolitology.com/health/anorexia.htm

[3] This discussion of the Ana movement draws on the following articles: Jill Barcum, "The Struggle with 'Ana,'" [Electronic version] *Minneapolis Star Tribune* (May 1, 2005); and Martha Irvine, "Worshipping 'Ana': Eating Disorders Take On a Life of Their Own for Sufferers," *Brainerd Daily Dispatch* (Tuesday May 31, 2005): 1A, 5A.

[4] www.nationaleatingdisorders.org

[6] Pamela Houston, "Out of Habit, I Start Apologizing," in *Minding the Body: Women Writers on Body and Soul,* ed., Foster (New York: Doubleday, 1994), 148.

[7] Quoted in Diana Eck, *A New Religious America: How a "Christian Country" Has Become the World's Most Religiously Diverse Nation* (Boston: 2001), 98.

[8] Serenity Young lists some of these examples in the "Introduction" of her *Anthology of Sacred Texts by and about Women*, ed. Young (New York: Crossroad, 1995), ix–xxviii.

[9] There are a number of excellent sources by Christian feminists who have exposed the myth that Christianity is inherently patriarchal. Two of the most important works about women's prominent role in the early church are by Elisabeth Schüssler Fiorenza: *In Memory of Her: A Feminist Reconstruction of Christian Origins* (New York: Crossroad, 1984) and *But She Said: Feminist Practices of Biblical Interpretation* (Boston: Beacon, 1992).

[10] Maura Kelly, "Hunger Striking," in *Going Hungry: Writers on Desire, Self-Denial, and Overcoming Anorexia,* ed. Kate Taylor (New York: Anchor books, 2008), 9.

[11] Kim Chernin, *The Obsession: Reflections on the Tyranny of Slenderness* (New York: Harper & Row, 1981), 100.

[12] Diana Eck makes this point in *Encountering God: A Spiritual Journey from Bozeman to Banaras* (Boston: Beacon, 1993), 155.

[13] Adapted from E. Kurtz and K. Ketcham, *The Spirituality of Imperfection: Storytelling and the Search for Meaning* (New York: Bantam, 2002), 145–146.

[14] P. S. Richards, R. K. Hardman, and M. E. Berrett, *Spiritual Approaches in the Treatment of Women with Eating Disorders* (Washington D.C.: American Psychological Association, 2007), 272–273.

[15] Pema Chödrön, *The Places That Scare You: A Guide to Fearlessness in Difficult Times* (Boston: Shambala, 2001), inside cover.

[16] Thich Nhat Hanh, *Peace Is Every Step: The Path of Mindfulness in Everyday Life* (New York: Bantam, 1992), 5

[17] Eck, *Encountering God*, 162.

[18] Susan Albers gives practical suggestions for practicing mindful eating in *Eating Mindfully: How to End Mindless Eating & Enjoy a Balanced Relationship with Food* (Oakland: New Harbinger, 2003).

[19] Eck, *Encountering God,* 120–123.

[20] Joan Chittister, *In Search of Belief* (Liguori: Liguori, 1999), 3.

[21] Marya Hornbacher, *Wasted,* 286.

2

FROM ILLUSION TO INSIGHT
Dispelling "The Myth of Thinness" and Creating a New Sense of Purpose

[1] Lois Banner, *American Beauty* (Chicago: University of Chicago Press, 1983), 5.

[2] These "beauty experts" are quoted in Banner, *American Beauty*, 106, 113.

[3] Roberta Pollack Seid, *Never Too Thin: Why Women Are at War With Their Bodies* (New York: Prentice Hall Press, 1989), 76.

[4] Tara Parker-Pope, "Better to Be Fat and Fit Than Skinny and Unfit." *New York Times*, August 18, 2008. Also, for a book that challenges our culture's assumption that being thinner is necessarily healthier, see G. A. Gaesser, *Big Fat Lies: The Truth about Your Weight and Your Health* (New York: Fawcett Columbine, 1996). For a book that explores the politics behind the so-called "obesity epidemic" in the United States, see J. Eric Oliver, *Fat Politics: The Real Story behind America's Obesity Epidemic* (New York: Oxford, 2005).

[5] Seid, *Never Too Thin*, 85–87.

[6] ibid, 148.

[7] ibid, 191, 201, 237–238.

[8] ibid, 107.

[9] ibid, 105–106.

[10] A good source for statistics and data regarding the economics of the diet industry is Laura Fraser, *Losing It! America's Obsession with Weight and the Industry that Feeds It* (New York: Dutton, 1997). For more recent projections about the weight loss industries' profits, see the report from Marketdata Enterprises, Inc. at: www.emaxhealth.com/69/11203.html

[11] This figure is from www.medialiteracy.com/stats_advertising.jsp.

[12] This is from biz.yahoo.com/e/080227/wtw10-k.html

[13] Michael Pollan, *In Defense of Food: An Eater's Manifesto* (New York: Penguin, 2008), 123–124, 150.

[14] Peg Tyre, "Getting Rid of Extra Pounds," *Newsweek* (Dec. 3, 2003): 61, 63.

[15] Michael Pollan, *The Omnivore's Dilemma: A Natural History of Four Meals* (New York: Penguin, 2006), p. 88–89.

[16] Kim Severson cites scientific studies that indict "high fructose corn syrup consumption as a major culprit in the nation's obesity crisis," pointing out that this "inexpensive sweetener flooded the American food supply in the early 1980s, just about the time the nation's obesity rate started its unprecedented climb." See "Sugar Coated: We're Drowning in High Fructose Corn Syrup. Do the Risks Go

beyond Our Waistline?" *San Francisco Chronicle* (February 18, 2004): E1. See also Michael Pollan, *In Defense of Food*, 122.

[17] Kim Severson, "Sugar Coated," E1. Percentage for the failure rate of commercial diets is cited in "Losing Weight: What Works, What Doesn't," *Consumer Reports* 58 (June 1993): 347–357.

[18] For more on diet industry figures, see the 2007 report by Marketdata Enterprises, Inc. at www.emaxhealth.com/69/11203.html. This is a reference to Morgan Sprulock's award-winning documentary film, *Super Size Me* (2004), which records the deleterious consequences of his experiment with eating all his meals at McDonald's for one month.

[19] As an example of the high-calorie meals at restaurants, nine of the breakfast meals listed on Denny's nutritional information document (available as a PDF on the website: www.dennys.com/LiveImages/enProductImage_473.PDF) contain over 1000 calories. The note about Americans eating 200 more calories per day than they did 10 years ago is from Craig Lambert's article: "The Way We Eat Now," *Harvard Magazine* 106:5 (May-June 2004): 51

[20] Dr. Henry Emmons, a psychiatrist at the University of Minnesota who incorporates holistic medicine and spirituality into his work with clients who suffer from depression, makes this point in his book, *The Chemistry of Joy: A Three-Step Program for Overcoming Depression through Western Science and Eastern Wisdom* (New York: Simon and Schuster) p. 92

[21] Jonathan Shaw, "The *Deadliest* Sin," *Harvard Magazine* 104:4 (March-April, 2004), 38.

[22] Juliet Schor reports on children's use of electronic media in *Born to Buy: The Commercialized Child and the New Consumer Culture* (New York: Scribner, 2004), 33. Gortmaker is quoted in Lambert, "The Way We Eat Now," 53.

[23] The National Institute on Media and the Family website: www.mediafamily.org.

[24] ibid.

[25] For the Fiji Islands study, see A. Becker, et al., "Eating Behaviours and Attitudes Following Prolonged Exposure to Television among Ethnic Fijian Adolescent Girls," *British Journal of Psychiatry* 180 (2002): 509–514. For the study on Arab adolescents, see N. Shuriquie, "Eating Disorders: A Transcultural Perspective," *Eastern Mediterranean Health Journal* 5:2 (1999): 354–360.

[26] Anita Arnand, *The Beauty Game* (New York: Penguin, 2002), 73–76, 188.

[27] I am grateful to Jenna McNallie and Emma Hoglund (my former students at Concordia College in Moorhead, MN) for their collaboration on a paper we researched and wrote together on this topic. The paper is entitled, "From California to Calcutta: Spreading the White-Western Devotion to Female Thinness—A Post-Colonial Feminist Analysis," which appears in the *Journal of Feminist Studies in Religion* 25:1 (Spring 2009): 19–41.

[28] Mervat Nasser, Melanie Katzman, and Richard Gordon (eds.), *Eating Disorders and Cultures in Transition* (New York: Brunner-Routledge, 2001), 3–11, 92–100.

[29] Abra F. Chernik, "The Body Politic," in *Listen Up: Voices from the Next Feminist Generation,* ed. Findlen (Seattle: Seal Press, 1995), 78.

[30] See Chapter 9 of Eckhart Tolle's *A New Earth: Awakening to Your Life's Purpose* (New York: Dutton, 2005).

[31] Thich Nhat Hanh, *For a Future to Be Possible: Buddhist Ethics for Everyday Life* (Berkeley, CA: Parallax Press, 2007), 11.

[32] This quote comes from Richard Rohr's article "Men's Journey to the True Self," which can be found at goliath.ecnext.com/coms2/gi_0199-6194566/Men-s-journey-to-the.html.

[33] Pema Chödrön, *Practicing Peace in Times of War* (Boston: Shambala, 2007), 46.

[34] This quote appears at the top of the www.mindonthemedia.org homepage (2008).

3

FROM IDOLATRY TO INSPIRATION
Seeing Through "The Icons of Thinness" and Finding New Sources for Self-Definition

[1] Margaret Miles, *Image as Insight: Visual Understanding in Western Christianity and Secular Culture* (Boston: Beacon, 1985), 7–9, 128.

[2] A. Field., et al., "Exposure to the Mass Media and Weight Concerns among Girls," *Pediatrics* 103:3 (March 1999): 660.

[3] Stanford and University of Massachusetts studies are cited by Jean Kilbourne in *Deadly Persuasion: Why Women and Girls Must Fight the Addictive Power of Advertising* (New York: The Free Press, 1999), 133. Other research on the negative effects of viewing media images includes T. K. Cash, et al., "Mirror, Mirror On the Wall? Contrast Effects and Self-Evaluation of Physical Attractiveness," *Personality and Social Psychology Bulletin* 9 (1983): 351–358; S. L. Turner, "The Influence of Fashion Magazines on the Body Image Satisfaction of College Women: An Exploratory Analysis 32 *Adolescence* (1997); N. Wartick, "Can Media Images Trigger Eating Disorders?" *American Health* 14 (1995): 26–27. For a discussion of the influence of young women's magazines on adolescent consumers, see Dawn Currie, *Girl Talk: Adolescent Magazines and Their Readers* (Toronto: University of Toronto, 1999).

[4] Margaret Miles discusses Ambrose's views in *Carnal Knowing: Female Nakedness and Religious Meaning in the Christian West* (Boston: Beacon, 1985), 92. Augustine's views are stated in his "Literal Commentary on Genesis," in *Women in the Early Church*, ed. E. Clark (Collegeville: Liturgical Press, 1983), 28–29, 40. According to Rosemary Radford Ruether, "maleness and spirituality are equated" within the

classical Christian tradition. See *Women and Redemption: A Theological History* (Minneapolis: Fortress, 1998), 5.

[5] Erasmus of Rotterdam, "The Handbook of The Militant Christian," in *The Essential Erasmus*, ed. and trans. J. Dolan (New York: New American Library, 1964), 29.

[6] Danzy Senna, "To Be Real," reprinted in *Women: Images and Realities, A Multicultural Anthology* (3rd Edition). Eds., Amy Kesselman, Lily McNair, Nancy Schneidenwind, (Boston: McGraw Hill, 2003), 54

[7] Melina Gerosa, "Diet Like A Man," *Ladies Home Journal* (September 1998): 146–147.

[8] "Reasonable Doubts," an interview with Katha Pollitt conducted by the *Women's Review of Books* 17:10–11 (July 2000): 11; "In the Corridors of Power," an interview with Lissa Mauscatine, Press Secretary to the First Lady [Hilary Clinton] conducted by the *Women's Review of Books* 17:10–11 (July 2000): 6.

[9] Maureen Dowd, "Should Obama Cover Up?" *New York Times* (March 7, 2009), accessed online at www.nytimes.com/2009/03/08/opinion/08dowd.html.

[10] See Eckart Tolle's discussion of "The Inner Body" in Chapter 6 of *The Power of Now: A Guide to Spiritual Enlightenment* (Novato, CA: Namaste Publishing, 1999), 107–127

[11] Mary Duenwald, "Body and Image: One Size Definitely Does Not Fit All [electronic version] *New York Times* (June 22, 2003).

[12] Juliet Corbett Heymeyer, *Religion in America*, Fourth Edition (Upper Saddle River: Prentice Hall, 2000), 2.

[13] Roberta Pollack Seid cites studies on the relationship between thinness and upward mobility in *Never Too Thin: Why Women Are at War with Their Bodies* (New York: Prentice Hall, 1989), 16. The prevalence of obesity in women of color and women who are poor is cited in P. Elmer-Dewitt, P., "Fat Times," *Time Magazine* (Jan. 6, 1996): 63. See also "Obesity in Minority Populations," American Obesity Association, AOA Facts Sheets (2002). On the various factors, including the societal injustices, contributing to higher levels of obesity among socially marginalized groups, see Angela Davis, "Sick and Tired of Being Sick and Tired: The Politics of Black Women's Health," *The Black Women's Health Book: Speaking for Ourselves*, ed. White (Seattle, WA: Seal Press, 1991), 18–26; Robyn McGee, *Hungry for More: A Keeping It Real Guide for Black Women on Weight and Body Image* (Seattle, WA: Seal Press, 2005), 12; and Beth MacInnis, "Fat Oppression" in *Consuming Passions: Feminist Approaches to Weight Preoccupation and Eating Disorders*, eds. Brown and Jaspers (Toronto: Second Story Press, 1993), 69–79.

[14] Becky Thompson, *A Hunger So Wide and So Deep* (Minneapolis: University of Minnesota Press, 1994), 44; 92.

[15] Lynn Mabel-Lois and Aldebaran, "Fat Women and Women's Fear of Fat," in *Shadow on a Tightrope: Writings by Women on Fat Oppression*, eds. Schoenfielder and Wieser (San Francisco: Spinsters/Aunt Lute, 1983), 52–57.

[16] Author bell hooks interprets the (relatively) increased inclusion of people of color in advertising as "the commodification of otherness," which she describes as one of patriarchal capitalism's techniques for spicing up "the dull dish that is mainstream white culture" in order to preserve its dominance. See hooks, *Black Looks: Race and Representation* (Boston: South End, 1992), 21.

[17] Marya Hornbacher, *Wasted: A Memoir of Anorexia and Bulimia* (New York: Harper-Flamingo, 1998), 229.

[18] Katherine Thanas, quoted in *Essential Zen*, eds. Tanahashi and Schneider (New York: HarperSanFrancisco, 1994), 34

[19] Carol Christ makes an interesting point that it is by *seeing* images of what we most value that what we deem sacred is revealed to us and becomes real for us. See *She Who Changes: Re-Imagining the Divine in the World* (New York: Palgrave, 2003), 227. Also, see Elisabeth Schüssler Fiorenza, *In Memory of Her: A Feminist Theological Reconstruction of Christian Origins* (New York: Crossroad, 1983) and Karen Torjensen, *When Women Were Priests: Women's Leadership in the Early Church and the Scandal of Their Subordination in the Rise of Christianity* (New York: HarperSanFrancisco, 1995).

[20] I am drawing here largely on the scholarship of Schüssler Fiorenza (*In Memory of Her)* and Torjensen (*When Women Were Priests).*

[21] See Sally Cunneen, *In Search of Mary: The Woman and the Symbol* (New York: Ballantine Books, 1996).

[22] Quoted in Sally Cunneen, *In Search of Mary*, p. 299.

[23] Diane Apostolos-Cappadona, *Encyclopedia of Women in Religious Art* (New York: Continuum, 1996), 48; Cunneen, 178.

[24] China Galland, *Longing for Darkness: Tara and the Black Madonna* (New York: Penguin, 1991).

[25] Bouthaina Shaaban, "The Muted Voices of Women Interpreters" reprinted in *Women and World Religions,* ed. L. J. Peach (Upper Saddle River, NJ: Prentice Hall, 2002), 279.

[26] Lucinda Joy Peach, "Women and Islam," in *Women and World Religions.* Ed. Peach, 251, 255; see also Margaret Smith, "Rabi'a the Mystic and her Fellow-Saints in Islam," reprinted in *Women and World Religions*, 271–278.

[27] Quoted in *Essential Sufism*, eds. James Faiman and Robert Frager, (New York: HarperSanFrancisco, 1997), 177.

[28] Judith Plaskow reinterprets the ancient legend of Lilith in "The Coming of Lilith: Toward a Feminist Theology," in *Womanspirit Rising: A Feminist Reader in Religion,* eds. Christ and Plaskow (New York: HarperSanFrancisco, 1979), 198–209. See also *Standing at Sinai*, p. 54.

[29] Susan Niditch, "Portrayals of Women in the Hebrew Bible," in *Women and World Religions*, 173.

30 Diana Eck discusses the "power" or "energy" of Shakti in *Encountering God: From Bozeman to Banaras* (Boston: Beacon, 1993), 136–137.

31 Eck, *Encountering God*, 141–142.

32 S. Boucher, *Kwan Yin: Buddhist Goddess of Compassion* (Boston: Beacon, 1999).

33 Carol Christ, "Why Women Need the Goddess: Phenomenological, Psychological, and Political Reflections," in *Womanspirit Rising: A Feminist Reader in Religion,* eds. Christ and Plaskow (New York: HarperSanFrancisco, 1979), 272–287.

34 Christ, *She Who Changes*, see especially 197–225.

4
FROM CONTROL TO CONNECTION
"The Rituals of Thinness" and Our Need for Transformation

1 Jenilee Hlavenka, "Health Related v. Appearance Related Reasons for Exercise: Which Encourages People to Maintain and Exercise Program?" *Community of Undergraduate Journals Online*, (Dec. 16, 2005) at cujo.clemson.edu/manuscript. php?manuscript_ID=118. See also M. Tiggemann and S. Williamson, "The Effect of Exercise on Body Satisfaction and Self-Esteem as a Function of Gender and Age, *Sex Roles: A Journal of Research* (July, 2000): 119–125; C. F. Zmijewski and M. O. Howard, "Exercise Dependence and Attitudes toward Eating in Young Adults," *Eating Behaviors* 4 (2003): 181–195; and A. Furnham, N. Badmin, and I. Sneade, "Body Image Dissatisfaction: Gender Differences in Eating Attitudes, Self-Esteem, and Reasons for Exercise," *The Journal of Psychology* (2002): 581–597.

2 The percentage of women who exercise to lose weight is based on a survey conducted by S. Wooley and O. Wooley in conjunction with *Glamour* magazine. See "Feeling Fat in a Thin Society," *Glamour* (Feb. 1984): 198–201.

3 Jean Kilbourne, "Still Killing Us Softly: Advertising and the Obsession with Thinness," in P. Fallon, M.A. Katzman, S.C. Wooley, eds., *Feminist Perspectives on Eating Disorders* (New York: Guilford Press, 1994), 395–418.

4 Diane Mickley, "Pregnancy and Eating Disorders," *Eating Disorders Today* 3:3 (2005): 6.

5 Plato, "Phaedo," excerpted in *Cooking, Eating, Thinking: Transformative Philosophies of Food*, eds. Curtin and Heldke (Bloomington: Indiana University Press, 1992), 25.

6 For a discussion of Paul's theology of the body, see Dale B. Martin, *The Corinthian Body* (New Haven: Yale University Press, 1995). Martin warns that we should not assume that terms such as "body" and "spirit" meant the same thing to ancient people as they do for Americans today (6–7). We must not read Paul through the lens of Cartesian dualism that many of us take for granted. Nevertheless, Paul's interpreters emphasized the dangers of physical desire. In *The Body and Society:*

Men, Women, and Sexual Renunciation in Early Christianity (New York: Columbia University Press, 1988), Peter Brown says that the Latin biblical scholar, Jerome, contributed significantly to a sexualized view of Paul's understanding of "the flesh." For Jerome, "an unrelieved sense of sexual danger, lodged deep within the physical person, swallowed up all other meanings of the flesh" (48, 276–277, 376). See also Theresa Shaw, *The Burden of the Flesh: Fasting and Sexuality in Early Christianity* (Minneapolis: Fortress, 1998).

[7] For a discussion of the ambiguous role of the body in Christian theology, see Lisa Isherwood and Elizabeth Stuart, *Introducing Body Theology* (Sheffield: Sheffield Academic Press, 1998), and Anne Spalding, "The Place of Human Bodiliness in Theology," *Feminist Theology* 20 (1998).

[8] According to Margaret Miles, the hierarchical tension between "body" and "soul" in early Christianity did not split into a radical dualism until the 17th century with the work of René Descartes. See *Fullness of Life: Historical Foundations for a New Asceticism* (Philadelphia: Westminster, 1981). Miles's work challenges the stereotypical assumption that early and Medieval Christian authors posited a radical separation between body and soul. Through a close and contextualized reading of primary Christian texts, Miles reconstructs a Christian history of ideas about the human body that underscores classical authors' assumptions that the human body and soul, though distinct, were inseparable. Although early Christian authors viewed the body and soul to be hierarchically ranked in an antagonistic relationship, they did not see them as ontologically or essentially separate, as Descartes later did.

[9] Starhawk, *Dreaming the Dark: Magic, Sex, and Politics* (Boston: Beacon, 1982), 1–14

[10] J. B. Vincent, "The Potential Value and Toxicity of Chromium Picolinate as a Nutritional Supplement, Weight Loss Agent and Muscle Development Agent," *Sports Medicine* 33:3 (2003): 213–230.

[11] S. Chaudhary, J. Pinkston, M. M. Rabile, and J. D. Van Horn, "Unusual Reactivity in a Commercial Chromium Supplement Compared to Baseline DNA Cleavage with Synthetic Chromium Complexes," *Journal of Inorganic Biochemistry* 99:3 (2005): 787–794.

[12] D. M. Stallings, D. D. Hepburn, M. Hannah, J. B. Vincent, J. O'Donnell, "Nutritional Supplement Chromium Picolinate Generates Chromosomal Aberrations and Impedes Progeny Development in Drosophila Melanogaster," *Mutation Research* 610:1–2 (2006): 101–113.

[13] D. D. Hepburn, J. Xiao, S. Bindom, J. B. Vincent, J. O'Donnell, "Nutritional Supplement Chromium Picolinate Causes Sterility and Lethal Mutations in Drosophila Melanogaster," *Proceedings of the National Academy of Science of the U.S.A.* 100:7 (2003): 3766–3771.

[14] See Expert Group on Vitamins and Minerals, "Risk Assessment: Chromium" (2003) at www.food.gov.uk/multimedia/pdfs/evm_chromium.pdf

[15] Several prominent historians of Christianity have noted the ironically central role of the body in Christian practices (especially asceticism) that appear to be based on bodily denial. According to Teresa Shaw, asceticism did not simply entail a dualistic rejection of the flesh but was engaged as a "strategy for empowerment and gratification." See *The Burden of the Flesh: Fasting and Sexuality in Early Christianity* (Minneapolis: Fortress, 1998), 6. See also Peter Brown, *The Body and Society*; Caroline Walker Bynum, *Holy Feast, Holy Fast: The Religious Significance of Food for Medieval Women* (Berkeley: University of California Press, 1987) and *Fragmentation and Redemption: Essays on Gender and the Human Body in Medieval Religion* (New York: Zone Books, 1991); Margaret Miles, *Practicing Christianity: Critical Perspectives for an Embodied Spirituality* (New York: Crossroad, 1988); and Sarah Coakley, ed. *Religion and the Body* (Cambridge: Cambridge University Press, 1997).

[16] Quoted in Jon Sweeney, *Praying with Our Hands: 21 Practices of Embodied Prayer from the World's Spiritual Traditions* (Woodstock: Skylight Paths, 2000), 20

[17] See Starhawk, *Dreaming the Dark*, 1–14.

[18] Christina Sell, *Yoga from the Inside Out: Making Peace with Your Body through Yoga* (Prescott: Hohm Press, 2003), 70.

[19] Christine Gorman reports on the Center for Disease Control study in "Is It O.K. to Be Pudgy?" *Time Magazine* (May 9, 2005): 47. On the health risks associated with aging and being underweight, see E. Kaldor and L. Closway, "Being Underweight Poses Health Risks," *Mayo Clinic Women's HealthSource* (May 2, 2005). See also Robyn McGee, *Hungry for More: A Keeping-It-Real Guide for Black Women on Weight and Body Image* (Emeryville: Seal Press, 2005), xxi; and Vivian F. Mayer, "The Fat Illusion," in *Shadow on a Tightrope: Writings by Women on Fat Oppression*, eds. Schoenfielder and Wieser, (San Francisco: Spinsters/Aunt Lute, 1983), 3–14.

[20] Rachel Wildman, Paul Muntner, et. al., "The Obese without Cardiometabloic Risk Factor Clustering and the Normal Weight with Cardiometabolic Risk Factor Clustering," *Archives of Internal Medicine* 168:15 (2008):1617–1624.

[21] Pat Lyons and Debora Burgard, *Great Shape: The First Fitness Guide for Large Women* (Lincoln, NE: iUniverse.com, Inc., 2000).

[22] The success of *Curves* is noted by Mary Duenwald in "Body and Image: One Size Definitely Does Not Fit All," [electronic version] *New York Times* (June 22, 2003).

[23] See K. Kratina, N. King, and D. Hayes, *Moving Away From Diets: New Ways to Heal Eating Problems and Exercise Resistance* (Lake Dallas: Helms Seminars Publishing, 1996). See Chapter 3 on "Joyful Movement," especially pp. 104–109.

[24] "Ruthie," quoted by Becky Thompson in *A Hunger So Wide and So Deep: American Women Speak Out on Eating Problems* (Minneapolis: University of Minnesota Press, 1994), 124.

[25] Anne Lamott, *Traveling Mercies: Some Thoughts on Faith* (New York: Pantheon Books, 1999), 197–198.

5

FROM JUDGMENT TO RESPONSIBILITY
"The Morality of Thinness" and Our Need for Virtue

[1] Margaret Miles points out that Eve, more than any other scriptural character in the Christian West, "was the basis for a fictional figure of 'woman' that allowed men to feel that they understood both the 'nature' of actual women and appropriate male roles and responsibilities in relation to women." See *Carnal Knowing: Female Nakedness and Religious Meaning in the Christian West* (Boston: Beacon, 1989), 119.

[3] Serenity Young, "Introduction," *An Anthology of Sacred Texts by and about Women*, ed., Young (New York: Crossroad, 1995), xx.

[4] See Rudolph Bell, *Holy Anorexia* (Chicago: University of Chicago Press, 1985).

[5] Caroline Walker Bynum, *Holy Feast and Holy Fast: The Religious Significance to Food for Medieval Women* (Berkeley: University of California Press, 1987). For a discussion of the term "anorexia mirabilis," see Joan Jacobs Brumberg, *Fasting Girls: The History of Anorexia Nervosa* (New York: Penguin, 1988).

[6] Quoted in Bynum, *Holy Feast and Holy Fast*, 168.

[7] In response to a religious authority who questioned the motives of her fasting, Catherine insisted that her inability to eat was an "infirmity," not a choice. See "Letter to a Certain Religious Person in Florence," *The Letters of Catherine of Siena*; Vol. 1, trans. and ed. S. Noffke (Binghampton: Medieval and Renaissance Texts and Studies, 1988), 79. On the other hand, Catherine's confessor, Raymond of Capua, interprets Catherine's fasting as proof of her supernatural holiness, insisting that "her whole life was a miracle." Raymond of Capua, *The Life of St. Catherine of Siena*, trans. G. Lamb (New York: P.J. Kennedy and Sons, 1960), 30–45, 51–59, 150–163.

[8] This is one of Bynum's key points in *Holy Feast and Holy Fast*. According to Bynum, food was a prominent religious symbol during the late Middle Ages due to its association with the Eucharist, but it was a particularly powerful symbol for women, who were typically involved in preparing and distributing food, and whose very bodies became food through the process of pregnancy and lactation. Fasting was thus central to late medieval women's asceticism (30, 191, 193). In Bynum's account, refusing to eat or digest food was not simply an expression of female self-hatred, or even a manifestation of body-hatred (218). Rather, the painful hunger that fasting engendered was a means for coming closer to God. Such pain connected a fasting woman with the suffering of Christ, and in so doing brought redemption to her and others (207). In this sense, medieval women's fasting practices also served as a means for spiritual self-definition. By abstaining from food to connect with God, women took spirituality into their own hands. Abstinence enabled ascetic women

to manipulate their environment as well. By refusing to eat or digest their food, they gained the adoration and recognition, and occasionally also the suspicion, of their peers (195). According to Teresa Shaw, early Church sources underscore the special importance of fasting for women. Women are reported to fast more rigorously than men, and they are encouraged to fast more often, despite occasional cautions by male authors against immoderate fasting. Shaw notes that some sources imply that women are better suited to fasting than men. In the words of one early Christian author: "It is fitting for women to fast always." Quoted in Shaw, *The Burden of the Flesh: Fasting and Sexuality in Early Christianity* (Minneapolis: Fortress Press, 1998), 233.

[9] In *The Burden of the Flesh*, Shaw discusses the meanings of ascetic women's emaciated bodies. The female ascetic's thin form, her withered breasts, the cessation of menstruation and the drying up of other reproductive fluids were seen as outward manifestations of inner purity. In the eyes of some Church Fathers, the destruction of sexual features among female ascetics helped counteract the power of attraction with which women were supposedly naturally endowed (to compensate for their lack of power in other realms). Thus the "deformity" of the female ascetic's skeletal, barren, dried up body was considered pleasing in the eyes of Church Fathers. John Chrysostom, for example, believed that the "beautiful state" of an ascetic woman's soul "is conferred upon her body." But the opposite was also true. For Chrysostom, nothing was more shameful and ugly than a gluttonous woman, stuffed full of food and drink. Such a woman was not only unhealthy but "rude," "slavish and thoroughly low-born" (133–135, 236).

[10] This point is similar to Bell's thesis in *Holy Anorexia*.

[11] Carolyn Costin, *Your Dieting Daughter: Is She Dying for Attention?* (New York: Brunner Mazel, 1997), 13.

[12] Hilde Bruch, *The Golden Cage: The Enigma of Anorexia Nervosa* (New York: Vintage, 1978), 58.

[13] Deborah Tolman and Elizabeth Debold, "Conflicts of Body and Image: Female Adolescents, Desire, and the No-Body Body," in *Feminist Perspectives on Eating Disorders,* eds. Fallon, Katzman, and Wooley (New York: Guilford, 1994), 307.

[14] Michael Pollan, *In Defense of Food: An Eater's Manifesto* (New York: Penguin, 2008), 1–2, 8, 10.

[15] R. Marie Griffith critically explores the Christian diet movement in *Born Again Bodies: Flesh and Spirit in American Christianity* (Berkeley: University of California Press, 2004), especially 160–250. My discussion of the movement draws heavily on Griffith's work.

[16] Griffith, *Born Again Bodies*, 177, 222

[17] ibid, 160–192.

[18] ibid, 180.

[19] Shelley Bovey, *The Forbidden Body: Why Being Fat is Not A Sin* (London: Pandora, 1989), 39, 49.

[20] Robyn McGee, *Hungry for More: A Keeping-It-Real Guide for Black Women on Weight and Body Image* (Seattle: Seal Press, 2005), 4–5.

[21] See www.cosmeticplasticsurgerystatistics.com/statistics.html#2007-HIGHLIGHTS.

[22] E. Dellinger Flum, "Impact of Gastric Bypass Operation on Survival: A Population-based Analysis, *Journal of the American College of Surgeons* 199: 4 (2004): 543–551.

[23] McGee, *Hungry for More*, 2–4.

[24] ibid, xix.

[25] M. Jocelyn Elders, "Foreword," *Hungry for More* by Robyn McGee, vii.

[26] Clifford Geertz makes this point in his classic essay, "Religion as a Cultural System," in his book *The Interpretation of Cultures* (New York: Basic Books, 1973), 95–97. To explore some alternative models of God, see Sallie McFague's *The Body of God: An Ecological Theology* (Minneapolis: Fortress, 1993) and her *Models of God: Theology for an Ecological, Nuclear Age* (Philadelphia: Fortress, 1987).

[27] Richard Strozzi Heckler, *The Anatomy of Change: A Way to Move Through Life's Transitions* (Berkeley: North Atlantic Books, 1993), xvi

[28] In 2005, the United Nations Food and Agriculture Organization (FAO) assessed the various significant impacts of the world's livestock sector on the environment. Its report, entitled *Livestock's Long Shadow: Environmental Issues and Options* documents the incredible damage that raising animals for food inflicts on the environment. See H. Steinfeld, et al., *Livestock's Long Shadow: Environmental Issues and Options* (available at www.fao.org/docrep/010/a0701e/a0701e00.htm).

[29] This concept and the exercise associated with it is based on Thich Nhat Hahn's mindfulness exercises in *The Miracle of Mindfulness: A Manual on Meditation* (Boston: Beacon Press, 1975).

[30] Pema Chödrön makes this point about the value of practicing pausing in *Practicing Peace in Times of War* (Boston: Shambala, 2007), 38–42.

[31] Eve Ensler, *The Good Body* (New York: Villard Books, 2004), 68–69.

[32] Quoted in Jon Sweeney, *Praying with Our Hands: 21 Practices of Embodied Prayer from the World's Spiritual Traditions* (Woodstock, VT: Skylight Paths, 2000), 49.

[33] Rich Pirog and Andrew Benjamin, "Checking the Food Odometer: Comparing Food Miles for Local Versus Conventional Produce Sales in Iowa Institutions," *Leopold Center for Sustainable Agriculture* (July 2003). See www.leopold.iastate.edu/pubs/staff/files/food_travel072103.pdf.

[34] Jane Goodall, *Harvest for Hope: A Guide to Mindful Eating* (New York: Warner Books, 2005), 285.

[35] Associated Press, "18,000 Children Die Every Day from Hunger, U.N. Says," *USA*

Today, 2/17/2007, accessed at: www.usatoday.com/news/world/2007-02-17-un-hunger_x.htm.

[36] L. Shannon Jung, *Food for Life: The Spirituality and Ethics of Eating* (Minneapolis: Fortress Press, 2004), 62, 78, 80.

[37] BAM is described by Alison Bass in "Anorexic Marketing Faces Boycott," *Boston Globe* (April 25, 1994): 1, 16.

[38] Kathy Bruin describes About Face in *Bitch* 3:2 (1998): 19–21.

[39] Ensler, *The Good Body*, 85–86.

6

FROM CONFORMITY TO SELF-ACCEPTANCE

"The Community of Thinness" and Our Need for Unconditional Love

[1] *Black Elk Speaks: Being the Life Story of a Holy Man of the Oglala Sioux*, as told through John Neidhardt (Lincoln: University of Nebraska, 1979 [1932]), 7.

[2] Mimi Nichter and Nancy Vuckovic, "Fat Talk: Body Image among Adolescent Girls," in *Many Mirrors: Body Image and Social Relations*, ed., Sault (New Brunswick: Rutgers University Press, 1994), 109–131.

[3] Linda Villarosa, "Dangerous Eating," *Essence* (January 1994): 18–21+.

[4] Becky Thompson, *A Hunger So Wide and So Deep: American Women Speak Out on Eating Problems* (Minneapolis: University of Minnesota Press, 1994). Some quantitative studies on the prevalence of eating problems among women of color include: F. Cacheline, E. Barzegarnazari, and R. H. Striegel-Moore, "Disordered Eating, Acculturation, and Treatment-Seeking in a Community Sample of Hispanic, Asian, Black, and White Women," *Psychology of Women Quarterly* 24 (2000): 244–253; R. H. Striegel-Moore, et al., "Drive for Thinness in Black and White Preadolescent Girls, *International Journal of Eating Disorders* 18:1 (1994): 59–69; D. Wilfley, et al., "Eating Disturbances and Body Image: A Comparison of a Community Sample of Adult Black and White Women," *International Journal of Eating Disorders* 20:4 (1995): 367–377; M. N. Miller and A. J. Pumariega, "Culture and Eating Disorders: A Historical and Cross-Cultural Review," *Psychiatry* 64:2 (2001): 93–110; L. W. Rosen et al., "Prevalence of Pathogenic Weight-Control Behaviors among Native American Women and Girls," *International Journal of Eating Disorders* 7 (1988): 807–811; L. Emmons, "Dieting and Purging Behavior in Black and White High School Students," *Journal of the American Diet Association* 92 (1992): 306–312; L. K. G. Hsu, "Are Eating Disorders Becoming More Common in Blacks?" *International Journal of Eating Disorders* 6 (1987): 113–124; T. J. Silber "Anorexia Nervosa in Blacks and Hispanics," *International Journal of*

Eating Disorders 5 (1986): 121–128; Maria Root, "Disordered Eating in Women of Color," *Sex Roles* 22 (1990): 525–536; J. E. Smith and J. Krejci, "Minorities Join the Majority: Eating Disturbances among Hispanic and Native American Youth," *International Journal of Eating Disorders* 10 (1991): 179–186; and L. Osvold and G. Sodowsky, "Eating Disorders of White American, Racial and Ethnic Minority American, and International Women," *Journal of Multicultural Counseling and Development* 21 (1993): 143–154.

[5] Retha Powers, "Fat Is a Black Woman's Issue," *Essence* (October, 1989): 75–78+.

[6] ibid.

[7] Marjory Nelson, "Fat and Old: Old and Fat," in *Shadow on a Tightrope: Writings by Women on Fat Oppression,* eds., Schoenfielder and Wieser (San Francisco, CA: Spinsters/Aunt Lute, 1983), 231.

[8] Pamela Houston, "Out of Habit, I Start Apologizing," in *Minding the Body: Women Writers on Body and Soul,* ed. P. Foster (New York: Doubleday), 150.

[9] Quoted in Pema Chödrön, *The Places That Scare You: A Guide to Fearlessness in Difficult Times* (Boston: Shambala, 2001), 9.

[10] Quoted in Matthew Fox, *Breakthrough: Meister Eckhart's Creation Spirituality in a New Translation* (New York: Doubleday, 1980), p. 99.

[11] Quoted in Diana Eck, *Encountering God: A Spiritual Journey from Bozeman to Banaras* (Boston: Beacon, 1993), xx.

[12] Thich Nhat Hanh relates and interprets this saying in *Living Buddha, Living Christ* (New York: Riverhead, 1995), 64.

[13] In her book, *The Millionth Circle*, Jean Shinoda Bolen suggests that when a critical number of people come together to support one another in changing their thinking and behavior, eventually the culture will follow and a new era will begin. Bolen offers guidance on both the practical and relational needs involved in creating circles that inspire personal and social transformation. *The Millionth Circle: How To Change Ourselves and the World* (Boston: Conari, 1999), 3. See also www.millionthcircle.com.

[14] See Kris Berggren, "Sharing the Journey of Spirit," *National Catholic Reporter* (May 26, 2006): 14–15.

[15] Eknath Eswaran, *The End of Sorrow: The Bhagavad Gita for Daily Living,* Volume 1 (Petaluma: Nilgiri Press, 1975), 54.

[16] This quote is mentioned on the webpage for Spiritual Directors International. See www.sdiworld.org/what_is_spiritual_direction2/what-is-islamic-spiritual-direction.html.

[17] See www.jonrobison.net/size.html.

[18] McGee, *Hungry for More*, 10, 43; Christy Haubeggar, "I'm Not Fat, I'm Latina," *Essence* (December 1994): 48.

[19] In *Sisters of the Yam: Black Women and Self-Recovery* (Boston: South End, 1993), the spiritually-grounded educator and cultural critic, bell hooks, demonstrates the transformative power of self-help communities of women of color. Though this book does not deal primarily with eating and body image problems, its discussions of topics like addiction, spirituality, work, truth-telling, eroticism, reconciliation, estrangement from nature (and more) are full of insights that pertain to the process of healing from disordered eating.

[20] Quoted in McGee, *Hungry for More*, 66–67.

[21] LoveMyBody is another organizational resource that promotes education and awareness about eating and body image problems among minority women. See www.lovemybody.org/index.cfm?zid=35&ContentID=1.

[22] Cheryl Townsend Gilkes, "The 'Loves' and 'Troubles' of African American Women's Bodies," in *A Troubling in My Soul: Womanist Perspectives on Evil and Suffering*, ed. Townes (New York: Orbis, 1993), 241.

[23] Jennifer Baumgardner and Amy Richards, *Manifesta: Young Women, Feminism, and the Future* (New York: Farrar, Straus, and Giroux, 2000), 6–7.

7
FROM ESCAPE TO PRESENCE
"The Salvation of Thinness" and Our Need for Peace

[1] These Native American views on "health" are presented in the film, *American Indian Concepts of Health and Unwellness* (1990), which is based on the 25-page monograph of the same title by Carol Locust, Ph.D.

[2] Paramahansa Yogananda, *Scientific Healing Affirmations: Theory and Practice of Concentration* (Los Angeles: Self-Realization Fellowship, 2003), 15.

[3] Thich Nhat Hanh, *Love In Action: Writings on Nonviolent Social Change* (Berkeley: Parallax Press, 1993), 70–71, 99.

[4] Lindsey Hall and Leigh Cohn, *Bulimia: A Guide to Recovery* (Carlsbad, CA: Gürze Books, 1999), 102.

[5] L. Shannon Jung, *Food for Life: The Spirituality and Ethics of Eating* (Minneapolis: Fortress Press, 2004), 6–8.

[6] Some good sources of information on women and work include: Arlie Hochschild, *The Second Shift: Working Parents and the Revolution at Home* (New York: Viking Penguin, 1989); Arlie R. Hochschild, *The Time Bind: When Work Becomes Home and Home Becomes Work* (New York: Metropolitan Books, 1997); Barbara Killinger, *Workacholics: The Respectable Addicts* (Buffalo: Firefly Books, 1991); Juliet Schor,

The Overworked America: The Unexpected Decline of Leisure (New York: Basic Books, 1991).

[7] David M. Levy uses the phrase "more-faster-better" to describe "a powerful philosophy that privileges 'fast-time' activities over 'slow-time' activities." See "No Time To Think: Reflections on Information Technology and Contemplative Scholarship," in *Ethics & Information Technology* 9:4 (2007): 237–249.

[8] Pema Chödrön, *The Places That Scare You: A Guide to Fearlessness in Difficult Times* (Boston: Shambala, 2001), 4, 50.

[9] Two qualitative studies that deal with the relationship between troubled eating and incest survival are Jennifer Manlowe's *Faith Born of Seduction: Sexual Trauma, Body Image, and Religion* (New York: New York University Press, 1995) and Becky Thompson's *A Hunger So Wide and So Deep: American Women Speak Out on Eating Problems* (Minneapolis: University of Minnesota Press, 1994). For a discussion of the controversy surrounding the status of the sexual abuse factor in the development of eating problems, see Susan Wooley, "Sexual Abuse and Eating Disorders: The Concealed Debate," in *Feminist Perspectives on Eating Disorders,* eds. Fallon, Katzman, and Wooley, (New York: Guilford, 1994), 171–211.

[10] This exercise was inspired by the following texts: Eckhart Tolle, *The Power of Now: A Guide to Spiritual Enlightenment* (Novato, CA; New World Library, 1999); Jon Kabat-Zinn, *Full Catastrophe Living: Using the Wisdom of Your Body and Mind to Face Stress, Pain, and Illness* (New York, Random House, 1990); Steve Hayes with Spencer Smith, *Get Out of Your Mind and Into Your Life* (Oakland, CA; New Harbinger Publications, 2005).

[11] Lynn Ginsburg and Mary Taylor, *What Are You Hungry For?: Women, Food and Spirituality* (New York, NY: St. Martin's Press, 2002), 5.

[12] Quoted in *Essential Sufism*, eds., Fadiman and Frager (New York: HarperSanFrancisco, 1997), 105.

[13] Eknath Eswaran, *The End of Sorrow: The Bhagavad Gita for Daily Living*, Volume 1 (Petaluma, CA: Nilgiri Press, 1975), 17; see also Diana Eck, *Encountering God: A Spiritual Journey from Bozeman to Banaras* (Boston: Beacon, 1993), 108–109.

[14] This is one of the basic messages of Yogananda's *Scientific Healing Affirmations*.

[15] Fadiman and Frager, eds., *Essential Sufism*, especially 14–17.

[16] Mihaly Csikszentmihalyi discusses the concept of "flow" in *Flow: The Psychology of Optimal Experience* (New York: HarperPerennial, 1990).

[17] Eve Ensler, *The Good Body* (New York: Villard Books, 2004), xv.

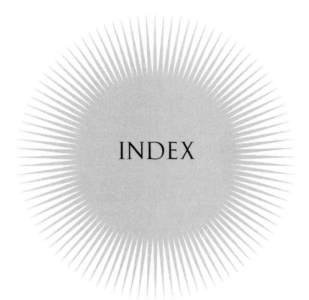

INDEX

ABOUT THE AUTHOR

In addition to *The Religion of Thinness*, Dr. Michelle Lelwica is also the author of *Starving for Salvation: The Spiritual Dimensions of Eating Problems among American Girls and Women* (Oxford, 1999), which is an academic analysis of the religious and cultural underpinnings of eating disorders and related problems. Additionally, she has published a number of scholarly articles, delivered papers, and lectured widely on the role of religion and spirituality in women's relationships with food and their bodies.

She is currently Associate Professor in the Religion Department at Concordia College—Moorhead, MN where she teaches classes that deal with embodiment, mindfulness, religion, gender, and cultural critique. She studied religion at Harvard Divinity School, where she received her Doctorate of Theology (ThD) in the area of Religion, Gender, and Culture in 1996.

Michelle lives with her husband and two children in northern Minnesota. She is motivated by the dream of creating a world in which the bodies and spirits of all people—and all beings—are loved, nurtured, and respected not in spite of but because of their marvelous diversity.

PRACTICING PEACE
WITH YOUR BODY

The concept of "practicing peace with your body" was introduced in the early stages of this book by Cissy Brady-Rogers, LMFT, an adjunct professor of Graduate Psychology at Azusa Pacific University and founder of Alive & Well Compassionate Health Coaching. She holds master's degrees in Theology and Marital & Family Therapy from Fuller Theological Seminary. A clinical member of the California Association for Marital & Family Therapy and the International Association of Eating Disorder Professionals, Cissy is also a certified spiritual director through the Claritas Institute for Interspiritual Inquiry and a certified yoga instructor.

In addition to psychotherapy, spiritual direction and health coaching services in Southern California, Cissy offers professional training on incorporating spirituality into clinical work and Practicing Peace with Your Body retreats, workshops, and groups.

For more information on these and other opportunities, please visit her website: *cissybradyrogers.com*.

ABOUT THE PUBLISHER

Since 1980, Gürze Books has been dedicated to providing quality information on topics related to eating disorders recovery, research, education, advocacy, and prevention. Thousands of professionals distribute their *Eating Disorders Resource Catalogue*, which is the most widely-used publication in this field, and Gürze has a variety of helpful websites including *www.bulimia.com* and *www.eatingdisordersblogs.com*.

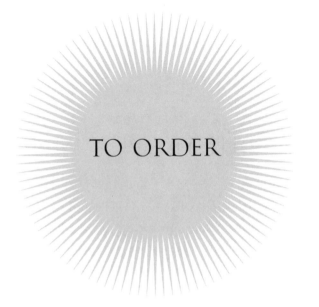

TO ORDER

Order additional copies of this book and find more information at *www.religionofthinness.com*. Quantity discounts are available from the publisher, Gürze Books, at (800)756-7533.

For book trade distribution, contact Publishers Group West/Perseus Book Group: *www.pgw.com*.